Atlas of
Human Anatomy on MRI
Spine Extremities Joints

Atlas of
Human Anatomy on MRI
Spine Extremities Joints

Hariqbal Singh MD DMRD

Professor and Head
Department of Radiology
Shrimati Kashibai Navale Medical College
Pune, Maharashtra, India

Parvez Sheik MBBS DMRE

Consultant Radiology
Department of Radiology
Shrimati Kashibai Navale Medical College
Pune, Maharashtra, India

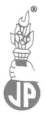

JAYPEE BROTHERS MEDICAL PUBLISHERS (P) LTD

New Delhi • St Louis • Panama City • London

Published by
Jaypee Brothers Medical Publishers (P) Ltd

Corporate Office
4838/24, Ansari Road, Daryaganj, **New Delhi** 110 002, India
Phone: +91-11-43574357, Fax: +91-11-43574314

Offices in India

- **Ahmedabad**, e-mail: ahmedabad@jaypeebrothers.com
- **Bengaluru**, e-mail: bangalore@jaypeebrothers.com
- **Chennai**, e-mail: chennai@jaypeebrothers.com
- **Delhi**, e-mail: jaypee@jaypeebrothers.com
- **Hyderabad**, e-mail: hyderabad@jaypeebrothers.com
- **Kochi**, e-mail: kochi@jaypeebrothers.com
- **Kolkata**, e-mail: kolkata@jaypeebrothers.com
- **Lucknow**, e-mail: lucknow@jaypeebrothers.com
- **Mumbai**, e-mail: mumbai@jaypeebrothers.com
- **Nagpur**, e-mail: nagpur@jaypeebrothers.com

Overseas Offices

- **North America Office, USA**, Ph: 001-636-6279734
  e-mail: jaypee@jaypeebrothers.com, anjulav@jaypeebrothers.com
- **Central America Office, Panama City, Panama**, Ph: 001-507-317-0160
  e-mail: cservice@jphmedical.com, Website: www.jphmedical.com
- **Europe Office, UK**, Ph: +44 (0) 2031708910 e-mail: info@jpmedpub.com

Atlas of Human Anatomy on MRI: Spine Extremities Joints

© 2011, Jaypee Brothers Medical Publishers

This book has been published in good faith that the material provided by authors is original. Every effort is made to ensure accuracy of material, but the publisher, printer and authors will not be held responsible for any inadvertent error(s). In case of any dispute, all legal matters are to be settled under Delhi jurisdiction only.

First Edition : 2011

ISBN 978-93-5025-233-8

Typeset at JPBMP typesetting unit

Printed at Replika Press Pvt. Ltd.

Whatever the mind of man can conceive and believe,
it can achieve

—Napoleon Hill

PREFACE

Human anatomy has not transformed but the advance in imaging modalities has changed the perception of structural details. With the advent of MRI, to know and understand the human anatomy is more important today than ever before. Thorough understanding of the normal MR anatomy is an essential prerequisite to precise diagnosis of pathology. MR imaging with its excellent resolution and multiplanar capability, helps in understanding complex anatomy and for this, the book is loaded with meticulously labeled illustrations.

It is steal a look into MR anatomy in an easy and understandable manner.

Atlas of Human Anatomy on MRI: Spine Extremities Joints will be extremely useful to undergraduates, residents in orthopedics and radiology, orthopedic surgeons, radiologists, general practitioners, other specialists, MRI technical staff and those who have a special interest in anatomy and imaging. It is meant for medical colleges, institutional and departmental libraries and for stand-alone MRI and orthopedic establishments.

Hariqbal Singh
Parvez Sheik

ACKNOWLEDGMENTS

We thank Prof MN Navale, Founder President, Sinhgad Technical Educational Society and Dr Arvind V Bhore, Dean, Smt Kashibai Navale Medical College for their kind acquiescence in this endeavor.

Our special thanks to the consultants Santosh Konde and Abhijit Pawar who have helped with their contributions in the book.

We profusely extend our gratefulness to the consultants Anand Kamat, Prashant Naik, Amol Sasane, Rahul Ranjan, Rajlaxmi Sharma, Sheetal Dhote, Dinesh Pardesi, Amol Nade, Manasi Bhujbal and Manisha Hadgaonkar for their genuine help in building up this educational entity.

Our appreciation for the CT and MRI technicians More Rahul, Demello Thomas, Musmade Bala and Raghvendra for their untiring help in retrieving the data.

Our gratitude to Manjusha Chikale, Nursing Sister; Snehal Nikalje, Anna Bansode and Sachin Babar for their clerical help.

We are grateful to God and mankind who have allowed us to have this wonderful experience.

CONTENTS

Plate 1

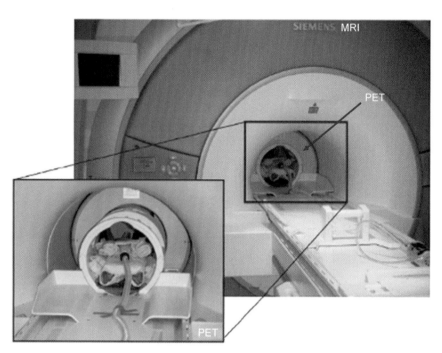

Fig. 15.1 MR-PET equipment, in this each scan occurs without repositioning the patient (*Courtesy:* Siemens Ag., Germany)

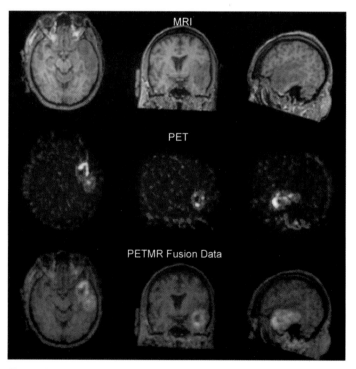

Fig. 15.2 MR-PET and fusion images demonstrates the glioma proliferation (*Courtesy:* Siemens Ag., Germany)

Plate 2

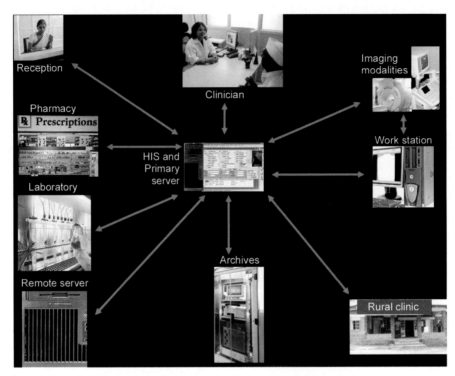

Fig. 16.1 Picture Archiving and Communication System (PACS) Flow chart

CHAPTER **1**

Physical Principle of Magnetic Resonance Imaging

Magnetic resonance imaging (MRI) is based on the principle of electromagnetic character of atomic nuclei which was first described by physicist Felix Bloch and Edward Purcell in 1946. They received a Noble prize for this in 1952. However, it was long after this that nuclear magnetic resonance was used for imaging. In 1973, Lauterbur showed that images of human body could be acquired by placing a magnetic field around it. First human images were published by Damadian et al in 1977. Since then use of MRI for medical imaging has seen an exponential growth and now it is a mainstay in the field of medical diagnostics.

Electromagnetism is at the core of MRI physics. When current is passed through a wire, a magnetic field is created around it. Similarly, in a nucleus with odd number of protons or neutrons, the electrons rotating around the nucleus produce a field around them. This gives a "charge" to the nucleus, also called as the spinning charge or "the spin". Thus these nuclei behave as tiny magnets. Hydrogen proton is the most favorable nucleus for MRI as it is widely available in the water molecules present in the body.

When these nuclei are placed in an external magnetic field (B_0), they either align along the magnetic field or against it. When the number of nuclei along the magnetic field is more as compared to those against the field, a net magnetization is created in the direction of the field.

In order to generate a signal from these spinning nuclei they have to be tipped out of alignment with B_0 (i.e. out of the longitudinal plane and towards the transverse plane). The signal generated by each rotating nucleus is much stronger if the nuclei precess in unison with each other at 90 degrees to the main magnetic field. For this a second magnetic field is introduced and it is referred to as B_1. This B_1 should be applied perpendicular to B_0, and it has to be at the resonant frequency. Radiofrequency (RF) coils are used to transmit B_1. If sufficient RF pulse is applied the spins are flipped into the transverse plane. This is the 90° RF pulse and it generates the strongest signal. However, as this is a high energy state, the signal starts decaying quickly and is called free induction decay (FID). This decay or relaxation is of two types:

T1 relaxation is the relaxation in the longitudinal plane due to the spins returning to the normal equilibrium state and aligning with the main magnetic field. In T2 relaxation there is dephasing in the transverse plane (90 degree plane). Each individual proton precesses at slightly different speed. After a while, the signal from protons in transverse plane degenerates as protons start precessing out of phase with each other. This is T2 relaxation.

In human tissue T1 is usually 10 times longer than T2 which means that T2 decay occurs before T1 recovery. In actual practice the T2 dephasing time is much quicker than the 'natural' T2 due to inhomogenities in the magnetic field B_0. This reduced T2 is called $T2^*$.

T1W and T2W images result by manipulating the manner and frequency in which RF pulses are applied (Repetition to Time), and by changing time to start signal acquisition after RF has been applied (Time to Echo), T1-weighted or T2-weighted images can be obtained.

Pulse sequences: (1) *Partial saturation (PS)*: It is also known as gradient echo or field echo and it uses a 90° RF pulse, (2) *Spin echo (SE)*: A 90° pulse is followed by 180° refocusing RF pulse. (3) *Inversion recovery (IR)*: 180° pulse is followed by a 90° pulse.

In a typical image acquisition, the basic unit of each sequence (i.e. the 90°-180° signal detection) is repeated hundreds of times. By altering the time to echo (TE) or time to repetition (TR), i.e. the time between successive 90° pulses, the signal contrast can be altered or weighted. For example, if a long TE is used, inherent differences in T2 times of tissues will become apparent. Tissues with a long T2 (e.g. water) will take longer to decay and their signal will be greater (or appear brighter in the image) than the signal from tissue with a short T2 (e.g. fat). In a similar manner TR governs T1 contrast. Tissue, with a long TR (water) will take a long time to recover back to the equilibrium magnetization value, therefore, a short TR interval will make this tissue appear dark compared to tissue with a short T1 (fat). When TE and TR are chosen to minimize both these weightings, the signal contrast is only derived from the number or density of spins in a given tissue. This image is said to be proton density weighted (PDW).

Air is black in all sequences because of very few protons and cortical bone is always black due to no mobility of protons.

Each volume element in the body has a different resonant frequency which depends on the protons present within it. This produces a signal which is specific to the resonant frequency of that volume element. This signal is analyzed by the computers using a mathematical technique called as Fourier analysis.

Magnet forms the main component of the MRI, it is of two types: (1) Permanent or resistive magnets used in low field scanners and are usually referred to as open MRI, (2) Superconducting magnet are used in all scanners above 1.0 Tesla. It is wound from an alloy (usually Nb-Ti) that has zero electrical resistance below a critical temperature. To maintain this temperature the magnet is enclosed and cooled by a cryogen containing liquid helium which has to be topped-up on a regular basis.

RF coils are needed to transmit and/or receive the MR signal. The RF coil should cover only the volume of interest. This gives an optimal signal-to-noise ratio (SNR). To achieve this there are various types of RF coils with trade-offs in terms of coverage and sensitivity, e.g. head coil being smaller in size provides better SNR. Body coil is integrated into the scanner bore and is not seen by the patient. Both these coils act as transceivers, i.e. they transmit and receive. Surface coils are used for imaging anatomy near to the coil. They are simple loop designs and have excellent SNR close to the coil but the sensitivity drops off rapidly with distance from the coil. These are only used as receivers, the body coil acting as the transmitter. Quadrature or circularly-polarized coils comprise of two coils 90° apart to improve SNR by a factor of $2^{1/2}$.

Advanced applications include diffusion imaging, perfusion imaging, functional MRI, spectroscopy, interventional MRI.

Possible adverse effects of **MRI** can be due to static magnetic field, gradients, RF heating, noise and claustrophobia.

Caution needs to be exercised while selecting patients for MRI. Patients with pacemakers, metallic implants, aneurysm clips should be excluded. Metallic objects should not be taken near the magnet as they can be injurious to the patient, personnel and equipment.

Special Sequences

Short Tau Inversion Recovery (STIR) Sequence

It is heavily T2 weighted imaging, as a result the fluid and edema return high signal intensity and it annuls out the signal from fat. The resultant images show the areas of pathology clearly. The sequence is useful in musculoskeletal imaging as it annuls the signal from normal fatty bone marrow.

Fluid Attenuated Inversion Recovery (FLAIR)

This is an inversion-recovery pulse sequence that suppresses or annuls out the signal from fluid/CSF. The sequence is useful to show subtle lesions in the brain and spinal cord as it annuls the signal from CSF. It is useful to bring out the periventricular hyperintense lesions, e.g. in multiple sclerosis.

Table 1.1	Time to echo and time to repetition for MR sequences		
	Time to Echo TE	**Time to Repetition TR**	
T1 weighted or T1W	Short TE	Short TR	
T2 weighted or T2W	Long TE	Long TR	
Proton density weighted or PDW	Short TE	Long TR	

Table 1.2	Signal intensity of various tissues at T1, T2 and proton density imaging		
Tissue	**T1**	**T2**	**Proton Density**
Fat	Bright	Bright (less than T1)	Bright
Water	Dark	Bright	Intermediate bright
Cerebral gray matter	Gray	Gray	Gray
Cerebral white matter	White	Dark	Dark
TR values	TR < 500	TR > 1500	TR > 1500
TE values	TE 50 to 100	TE > 80	TE < 50

Gradient Echo Sequence

This sequence reduces the scan times. This is achieved by giving a shorter RF pulse leading to a lesser amount of disruption to the magnetic vectors. The sequence is useful in identifying calcification and blood degradation products.

Diffusion-Weighted Imaging

'Diffusion' portrays the movement of molecules due to random motion. It enables to distinguish between rapid diffusion of protons (unrestricted diffusion) and slow diffusion of protons (restricted diffusion). GRE pulse sequence has been devised to image the diffusion of water through tissues. It is a sensitive way of detecting acute brain infarcts, where diffusion is reduced or restricted.

MR Angiography

The most common MR angiographic techniques are time-of-flight imaging and phase contrast. In these sequences, multiple RF pulses are applied with short TRs saturate the spins in stationary tissues. This results in suppression of the signal from stationary tissues in the imaging slab. In-flowing blood is unaffected by the repetitive RF pulses, as a result, as it enters the imaging slab, its signal is not suppressed and appears hyperintense compared with that of stationary tissue. Time-of-flight imaging may be 2D, with section-by-section acquisition, or 3D, with acquisition of a larger volume. Dynamic MRA can also be performed with intravenous gadolinium when in the vascular phase of enhancement.

CHAPTER **2**

Spine

The spine is made up of five groups of vertebrae. The portion of spine around the neck region is cervical spine. It is formed by first seven vertebrae which are referred as C1 to C7. Followed by twelve thoracic vertebrae, i.e. T1 to T12 and subsequently five lumbar vertebrae L1 to L5 in the low back area. The sacrum is a big triangular bone at the base, its broad upper part joins the L5 vertebra and its narrow lower part joins the coccyx or tail bone.

Cervical spine: It starts with first cervical vertebra (C1) attached to the bottom of the skull. First vertebra or C1 is called, atlas as it supports and balances the weight of the skull. It has practically no body or spinous process, it appears as two thickened bony arches to form a large hole with two transverse processes. On its upper surface, the atlas has two facets that unite with the occipital condyles of the skull. Structure of atlas is unique and has a large opening which accommodates spinal cord which is widest here.

The second vertebra is the "axis", it lies directly beneath the atlas vertebra. It bears large bony tooth-like protrusion on its summit, the odontoid process or the dens. This process projects upward and lies in the ring of the atlas. The joints of the axis give the neck its ability to turn from side to side i.e. left and right, as the head is turned, the atlas pivots around the odontoid process.

The transverse processes of the cervical vertebrae are distinctive because they have transverse foramina, which serve as passageways for vertebral arteries leading to the brain. Also, the spinous processes of the second to fifth cervical vertebrae are forked providing attachments for various muscles.

C3-C6 vertebrae have a typical structure. C7 vertebra is called vertebra prominens because of a long prominent thick nearly horizontal not bifurcated spinous process which is palpable from the skin.

Neural foramina of cervical spine allow way out to cervical spinal nerves which are eight in number and are named as C1 to C8.

Thoracic spine: It consists of twelve vertebrae in the chest area, the first thoracic vertebra articulates with the C7 vertebra above and the last thoracic vertebra articulates with the first

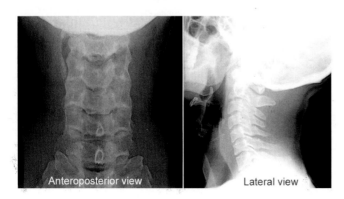

Anteroposterior view   Lateral view   **Fig. 2.1** Cervical spine

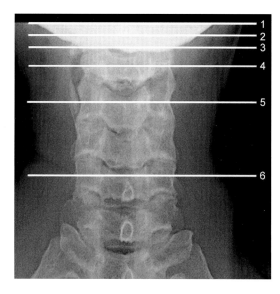

Fig. 2.2 Cervical spine MRI: Axial section plan

lumbar vertebra below. The thoracic vertebrae are larger in size than those in the cervical region. They have long, pointed spinous processes that slope downward, and have facets on the sides of their bodies that join with ribs. From the third thoracic vertebra onwards to the last thoracic vertebra, the bodies of these bones increases in size gradually. This reflects the stress placed on them by the increasing amounts of body weight they bear.

Lumbar spine: There are five "lumbar vertebrae" in the lower back. They have larger and stronger bodies to provide support.

The transverse processes of these vertebrae project backward at sharp angles, while their short, thick spinous processes are directed nearly horizontally.

Sacrum: The sacrum is a large triangular bone at the base of the lower spine. Its broad upper part joins the lowest lumbar vertebrae and its narrow lower part joins the coccyx or "tail bone". The sides are connected to the iliac bones (the largest bones forming the pelvis). The sacrum is a strong bone and rarely fractures. The five vertebrae that make up the sacrum are separate in early life, but gradually become

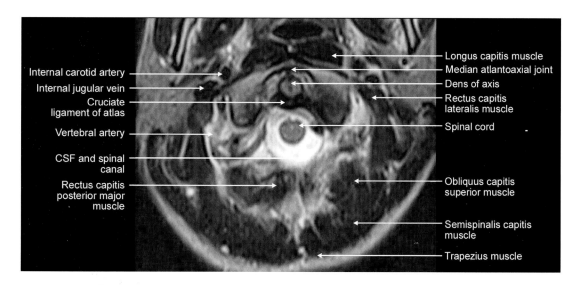

Fig. 2.3 Cervical spine MRI: Axial T2WI level at C1 (corresponds to level 1 in Fig. 2.2)

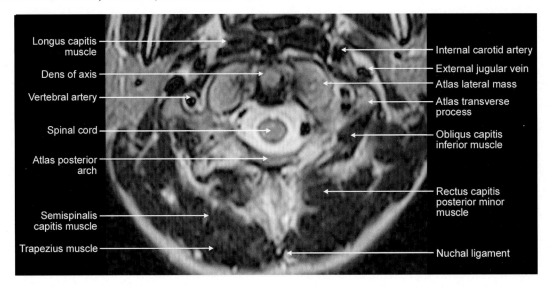

Fig. 2.4 Cervical spine MRI: Axial T2WI at level upper part of C2 vertebra (corresponds to level 2 in Fig. 2.2)

fused between the eighteenth and thirtieth years. The spinous processes of these fused bones are represented by a ridge of tubercles. The weight of the body is transmitted to the legs through the pelvic girdle at these joints.

Coccyx: It is the lowest part of the vertebral column and is attached by ligaments to the margins of the sacral hiatus. When a person is sitting, pressure is exerted on the coccyx, and it moves forward, acting like a shock absorber. Sitting down with force may cause the coccyx to be fractured or dislocated.

General features of spine: The vertebral body is shaped like an hourglass, thinner in the center with thicker ends. Outer cortical bone extends above and below the superior and inferior ends of the vertebrae to form rims. The superior and inferior endplates are contained within these rims of bone. The bodies of adjacent vertebrae are joined on the front surfaces by "anterior ligaments" and on the back by "posterior ligaments". A longitudinal row of the bodies supports the weight of the head and trunk.

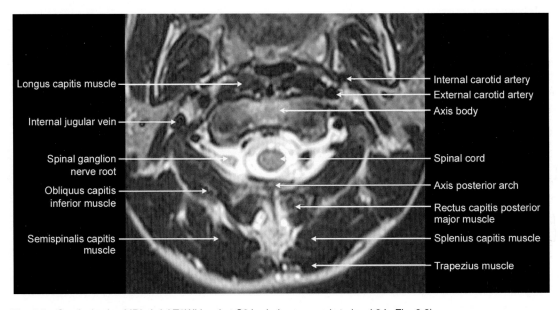

Fig. 2.5 Cervical spine MRI: Axial T2WI level at C2 body (corresponds to level 3 in Fig. 2.2)

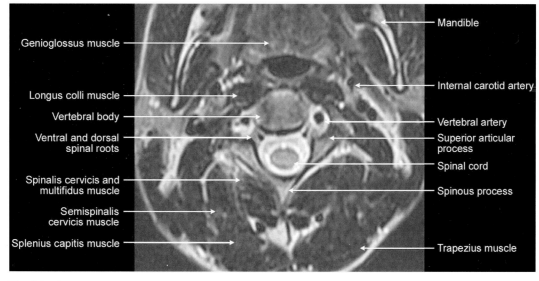

Fig. 2.6 Cervical spine MRI: Axial T2WI at C3 level (corresponds to level 4 in Fig. 2.2)

The anterior longitudinal ligament is a flat band that extends from the basiocciput of the skull and the anterior tubercle of the atlas to the front of the upper part of the sacrum. It is attached to the periosteum of the underlying vertebral bodies.

The posterior longitudinal ligament extends from the back of the body of axis to the anterior wall of the upper sacral canal.

Intervertebral disks are found between each vertebra. Intervertebral disks make up about one-third of the length of the spine and constitute the largest organ in the body without its own blood supply. The disks receive their blood supply through movement. The disks are flat, round structures about a quarter to three quarters of an inch thick with tough outer rings of tissue called the annulus fibrosis that contain a soft, white, jelly-like center called the nucleus pulposus. Flat,

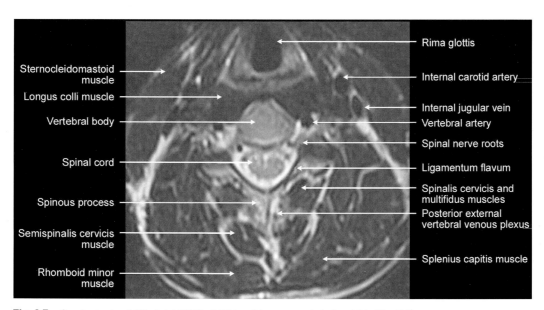

Fig. 2.7 Cervical spine MRI: Axial T2WI at C4 level (corresponds to level 5 in Fig. 2.2)

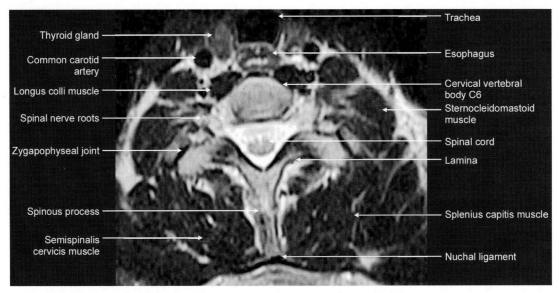

Thyroid gland

Common carotid artery

Longus colli muscle

Spinal nerve roots

Zygapophyseal joint

Spinous process

Semispinalis cervicis muscle

Trachea

Esophagus

Cervical vertebral body C6

Sternocleidomastoid muscle

Spinal cord

Lamina

Splenius capitis muscle

Nuchal ligament

Fig. 2.8 Cervical spine MRI: Axial at T2WI C6 level (corresponds to level 6 in Fig. 2.2)

circular plates of cartilage connect to the vertebrae above and below each disk. Intervertebral disks separate the vertebrae, but they act as shock absorbers for the spine.

Projecting from the back of each body of the vertebra are two short rounded stalks called "pedicles". They form the sides of the "vertebral foramen". They extend posteriorly from the lateral margin of the dorsal surface of the vertebral body.

The laminae are two flattened plates of bone extending medially from the pedicles to form the posterior wall of the

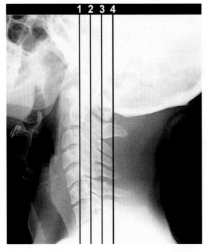

Fig. 2.9 Cervical spine MRI: Coronal section plan

vertebral foramen. They fuse in the back to become spinous process. The pars interarticularis is a special region of the lamina between the superior and inferior articular processes. A fracture or congenital anomaly of the pars may result in a spondylolisthesis.

The pedicles, laminae, and spinous process together complete a bony vertebral arch around the vertebral opening, through which the spinal cord passes. Between the pedicles and laminae of a typical vertebra is a "transverse process" that projects laterally and toward the back. Various ligaments and muscles are attached to the transverse process. Projecting upward and downward from each vertebral arch are "superior" and "inferior" articulating processes. These processes bear cartilage-covered facets by which each vertebra is joined to the one above and the one below it. These facet joints facilitate smooth gliding movement of one vertebra on another to produce twisting motions and rotation of the spine. Facet joints are also called as zygapophyseal joints.

On the surfaces of the vertebral pedicles are notches that align to create openings, called "intervertebral foramina". These openings provide passageways for spinal nerves that exit out of the spinal cord.

The ligamentum flavum is a strong ligament that connects the laminae of the vertebrae. The ligamentum flavum serves to protect the neural elements and the spinal cord and stabilize the spine so that excessive motion between the vertebral bodies does not occur. It is the strongest of the spinal ligaments and often has a thinner middle section. Together with the laminae, it forms the posterior wall of the spinal canal.

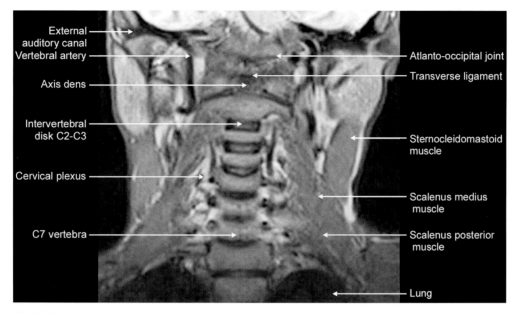

External auditory canal
Vertebral artery
Axis dens
Intervertebral disk C2-C3
Cervical plexus
C7 vertebra

Atlanto-occipital joint
Transverse ligament
Sternocleidomastoid muscle
Scalenus medius muscle
Scalenus posterior muscle
Lung

Fig. 2.10 Cervical spine MRI: Coronal T2WI (corresponds to level 1 in Fig. 2.9)

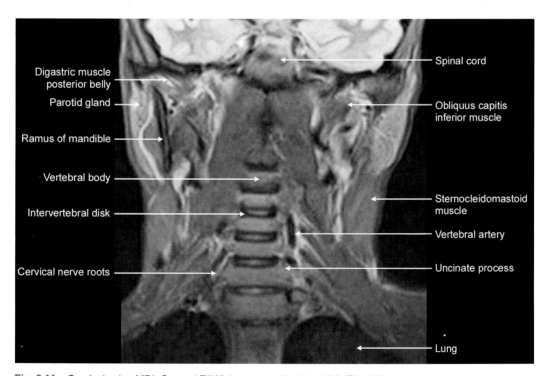

Digastric muscle posterior belly
Parotid gland
Ramus of mandible
Vertebral body
Intervertebral disk
Cervical nerve roots

Spinal cord
Obliquus capitis inferior muscle
Sternocleidomastoid muscle
Vertebral artery
Uncinate process
Lung

Fig. 2.11 Cervical spine MRI: Coronal T2WI (corresponds to level 2 in Fig. 2.9)

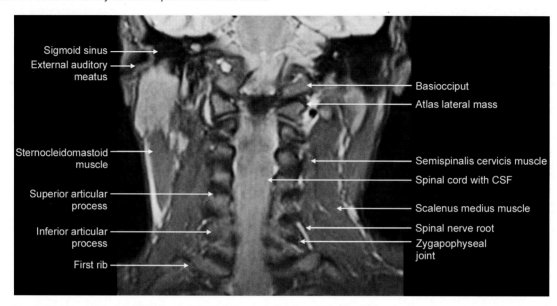

Sigmoid sinus

External auditory meatus

Basiocciput

Atlas lateral mass

Sternocleidomastoid muscle

Semispinalis cervicis muscle

Spinal cord with CSF

Superior articular process

Scalenus medius muscle

Inferior articular process

Spinal nerve root

Zygapophyseal joint

First rib

Fig. 2.12 Cervical spine MRI: Coronal T2WI (corresponds to level 3 in Fig. 2.9)

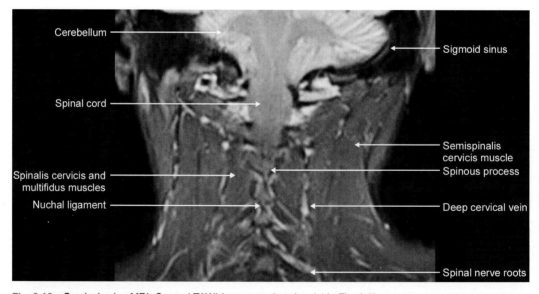

Cerebellum

Sigmoid sinus

Spinal cord

Semispinalis cervicis muscle

Spinous process

Spinalis cervicis and multifidus muscles

Nuchal ligament

Deep cervical vein

Spinal nerve roots

Fig. 2.13 Cervical spine MRI: Coronal T2WI (corresponds to level 4 in Fig. 2.9)

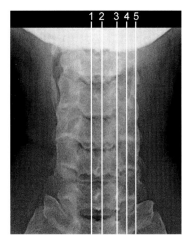

Fig. 2.14 Cervical spine: Sagittal section plan

Supraspinous ligaments join the tips of adjacent spinous process in the dorsal spine. In the neck they are replaced by the ligamentum nuchae and they are poorly developed in the lumbar region. During full flexion these ligaments are taut and support the spine. Interspinous ligaments are well developed only in the lumbar region, uniting the spinous process along their adjacent borders. Intertransverse ligaments join the tranverse processes along their adjacent borders.

Accessory ligaments: These connect the axis to the occiput, bypassing the atlas. They are the tectorial membrane, cruciform ligament, apical ligament and the paired alar ligaments.

Spinal canal: It is closed anteriorly by the vertebral bodies, the intervertebral disks, posterior longitudinal ligament. Posteriorly it is related to the lamina and ligamentum flavum. Laterally on either sides it is related to the pedicles. The intervertebral foramina contain the spinal nerves, posterior root ganglia spinal arteries and veins. The vertebral canal contains the spinal cord.

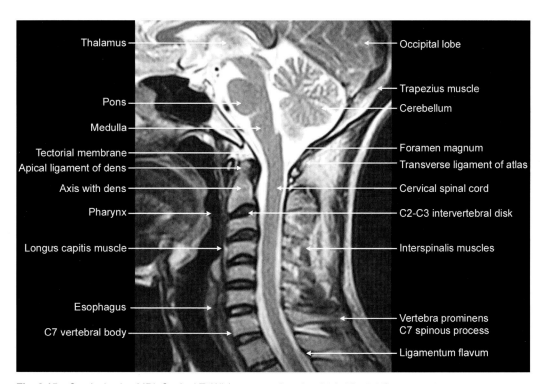

Fig. 2.15 Cervical spine MRI: Sagittal T2WI (corresponds to level 1 in Fig. 2.14)

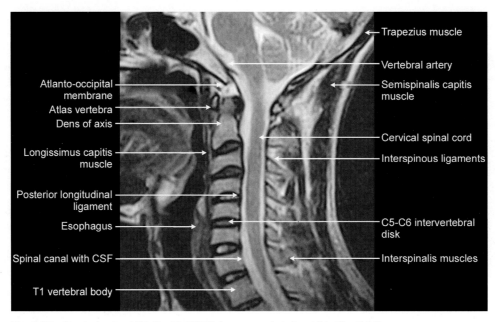

Atlanto-occipital membrane

Atlas vertebra

Dens of axis

Longissimus capitis muscle

Posterior longitudinal ligament

Esophagus

Spinal canal with CSF

T1 vertebral body

Trapezius muscle

Vertebral artery

Semispinalis capitis muscle

Cervical spinal cord

Interspinous ligaments

C5-C6 intervertebral disk

Interspinalis muscles

Fig. 2.16 Cervical spine MRI: Sagittal T2WI (corresponds to level 2 in Fig. 2.14)

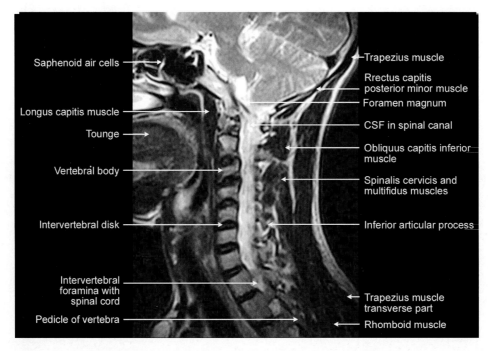

Saphenoid air cells

Longus capitis muscle

Tounge

Vertebral body

Intervertebral disk

Intervertebral foramina with spinal cord

Pedicle of vertebra

Trapezius muscle

Rrectus capitis posterior minor muscle

Foramen magnum

CSF in spinal canal

Obliquus capitis inferior muscle

Spinalis cervicis and multifidus muscles

Inferior articular process

Trapezius muscle transverse part

Rhomboid muscle

Fig. 2.17 Cervical spine MRI: Sagittal T2WI (corresponds to level 3 in Fig. 2.14)

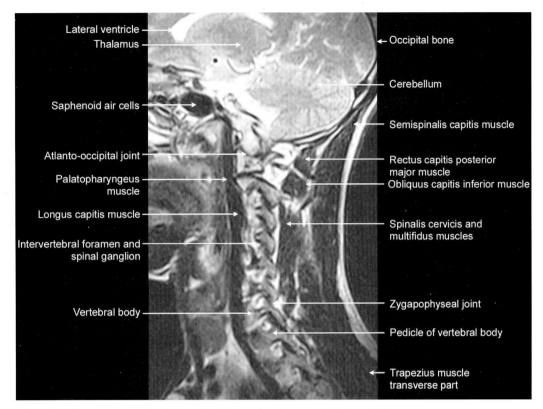

Lateral ventricle —
Thalamus —
— Occipital bone

— Cerebellum

Saphenoid air cells —
— Semispinalis capitis muscle

Atlanto-occipital joint —
— Rectus capitis posterior major muscle
Palatopharyngeus muscle —
— Obliquus capitis inferior muscle
Longus capitis muscle —
Intervertebral foramen and spinal ganglion —
— Spinalis cervicis and multifidus muscles

Vertebral body —
— Zygapophyseal joint

— Pedicle of vertebral body

— Trapezius muscle transverse part

Fig. 2.18 Cervical spine MRI: Sagittal T2WI (corresponds to level 4 in Fig. 2.14)

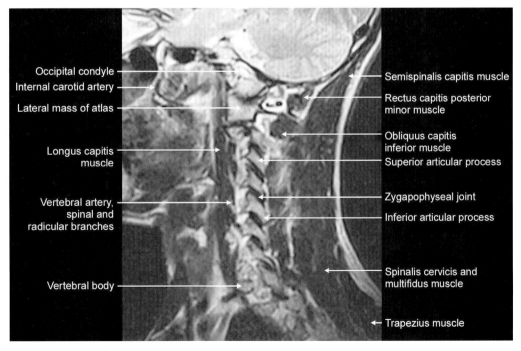

Occipital condyle —
Internal carotid artery —
— Semispinalis capitis muscle
Lateral mass of atlas —
— Rectus capitis posterior minor muscle

— Obliquus capitis inferior muscle
Longus capitis muscle —
— Superior articular process

Vertebral artery, spinal and radicular branches —
— Zygapophyseal joint

— Inferior articular process

— Spinalis cervicis and multifidus muscle

Vertebral body —
— Trapezius muscle

Fig. 2.19 Cervical spine MRI: Sagittal T2WI (corresponds to level 5 in Fig. 2.14)

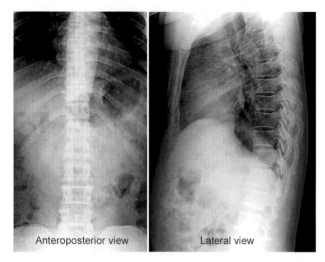

Anteroposterior view   Lateral view

Fig. 2.20   Dorsal spine

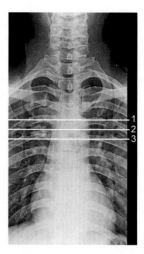

Fig. 2.21   Dorsal spine: Axial section plan

The spinal cord: The spinal canal encases the spinal cord. The bones and ligaments of the spinal column are aligned in such a manner to create a column that provides protection and support for the spinal cord. The outermost layer that surround the spinal cord is the dura mater, which is a tough membrane that encloses the spinal cord and prevents cerebrospinal fluid from leaking out. The space between the dura and the spinal canal is called the epidural space. This space is filled with tissue, vessels and large veins. The spinal cord is derived from the ectodermal neural groove, which eventually closes to form a tube during fetal development. From this neural tube, the entire central nervous system, eventually develops. Up to the third month of fetal life, the spinal

cord is about the same length as the canal. The growth of the canal outpaces that of the cord from the 3rd month onwards. In an adult the lower end of the spinal cord usually ends at approximately the first lumbar vertebra, where it divides into many individual nerve roots that travel to the lower body and legs. This collection of group of nerve roots is called the "cauda equina".

Some differentiating features between cervical, thoracic and lumbar vertebrae: C3-C6 vertebrae have atypical features. The body of these four vertebrae is small and broader from side-to-side than from front-to-back. The pedicles are directed laterally and backward. The laminae are narrow, and thinner above than below. The vertebral foramen is large and has a

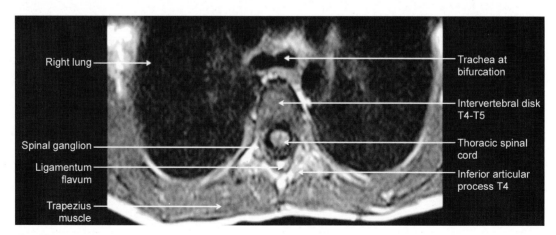

Right lung

Spinal ganglion

Ligamentum flavum

Trapezius muscle

Trachea at bifurcation

Intervertebral disk T4-T5

Thoracic spinal cord

Inferior articular process T4

Fig. 2.22   Dorsal spine MRI: Axial T1WI at level D4-D5 disk (corresponds to level 1 in Fig. 2.21)

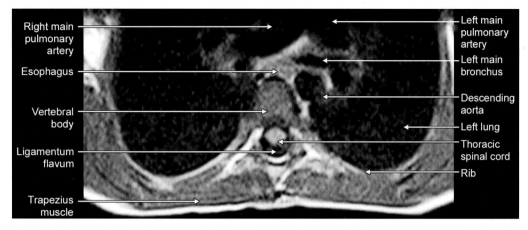

Right main pulmonary artery

Esophagus

Vertebral body

Ligamentum flavum

Trapezius muscle

Left main pulmonary artery

Left main bronchus

Descending aorta

Left lung

Thoracic spinal cord

Rib

Fig. 2.23 Dorsal spine MRI: Axial T1WI at level D5 lower part vertebral body (corresponds to level 3 in Fig. 2.21)

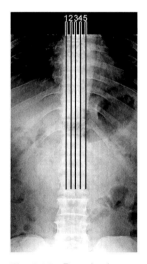

Fig. 2.24 Dorsal spine: Sagittal section plan

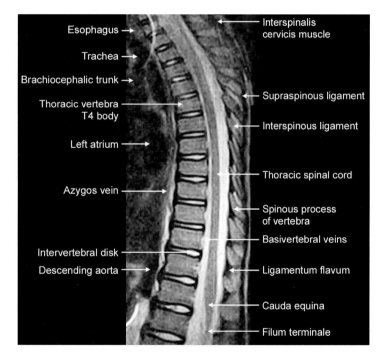

Esophagus

Trachea

Brachiocephalic trunk

Thoracic vertebra T4 body

Left atrium

Azygos vein

Intervertebral disk

Descending aorta

Interspinalis cervicis muscle

Supraspinous ligament

Interspinous ligament

Thoracic spinal cord

Spinous process of vertebra

Basivertebral veins

Ligamentum flavum

Cauda equina

Filum terminale

Fig. 2.25 Dorsal spine MRI: Sagittal T2WI (corresponds to level 1 in Fig. 2.24)

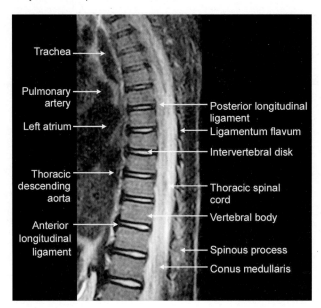

Fig. 2.26 Dorsal spine MRI: Sagittal T2WI (corresponds to level 2 in Fig. 2.24)

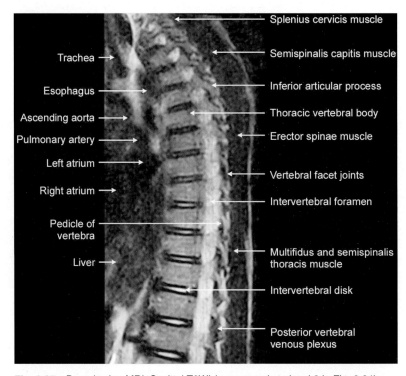

Fig. 2.27 Dorsal spine MRI: Sagittal T2WI (corresponds to level 3 in Fig. 2.24)

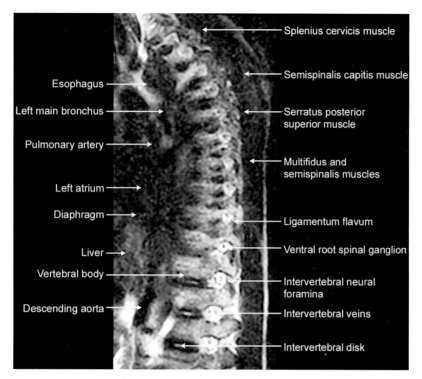

Fig. 2.28 Dorsal spine MRI: Sagittal T2WI (corresponds to level 4 in Fig. 2.24)

triangular shape. The spinous process is short and bifid. Superior articular facets face backward, upward, and slightly medially and inferior face forward, downward, and slightly laterally. The **foramen transversarium** is the openings in the transverse processes of the seven cervical vertebrae. It gives passage to the vertebral artery, vein and plexus of sympathetic nerves in each of the vertebrae except the seventh, which lacks the artery. C7 has enlarged spinous process called the vertebral prominence.

The thoracic vertebrae have costal facets for ribs on either sides of the vertebral body. They increase in size gradually from T3 vertebra downwards.

The lumbar vertebrae have neither a foramen in transverse process nor costal facets; they are also larger than the dorsal and cervical vertebrae in size.

Radiological importance of vertebral column in spinal injuries: The vertebral column can be subdivided as anterior column, middle column and the posterior column. Injuries involving the middle and posterior columns result in unstable injuries.

1. Anterior column is formed by anterior longitudinal ligament, anterior annulus fibrosus and anterior part of vertebral body.
2. Middle column is formed by posterior longitudinal ligament, posterior annulus fibrosus and posterior part of vertebral body.
3. Posterior column includes posterior elements and ligaments.

Radiological importance of craniovertebral junction: Chamberlain line is the line between posterior part of hard palate and posterior margin of foramen magnum. Normally the tip of odontoid process lies at or below this line. **Basilar line** is the line along the clivus and it usually falls tangent to posterior aspect of tip of odontoid.

Craniovertebral angle (Clivus-Canal angle) is angle between basilar line and a line along posterior aspect of odontoid process. If this angle is < 150°, cord compression can occur on the ventral aspect.

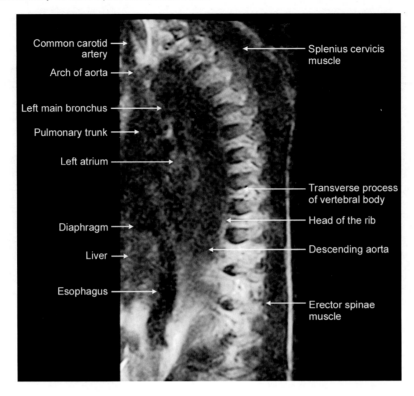

Common carotid artery
Arch of aorta
Left main bronchus
Pulmonary trunk
Left atrium
Diaphragm
Liver
Esophagus

Splenius cervicis muscle
Transverse process of vertebral body
Head of the rib
Descending aorta
Erector spinae muscle

Fig. 2.29   Dorsal spine MRI: Sagittal T2WI (corresponds to level 5 in Fig. 2.24)

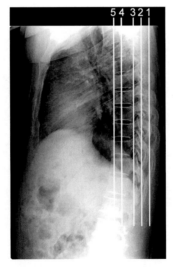

Fig. 2.30   Dorsal spine: Coronal section plan

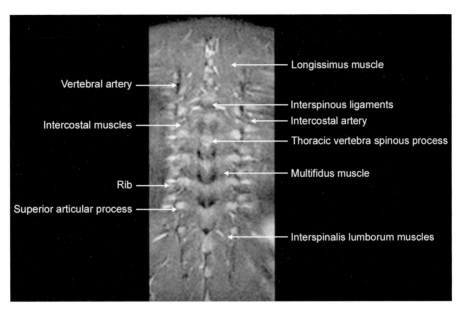

Fig. 2.31 Dorsal spine MRI: Coronal T2WI (corresponds to level 1 in Fig. 2.30)

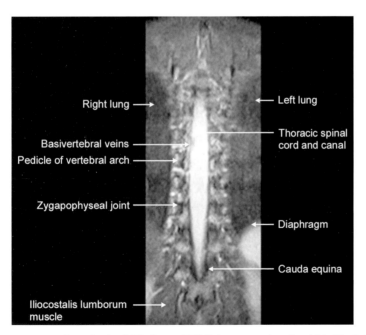

Fig. 2.32 Dorsal spine MRI: Coronal T2WI (corresponds to level 2 in Fig. 2.30)

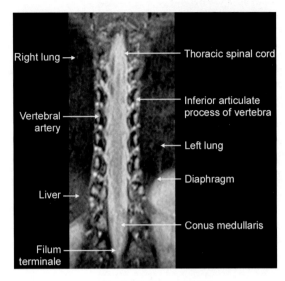

Right lung →

Thoracic spinal cord

Inferior articulate process of vertebra

Vertebral artery

Left lung

Diaphragm

Liver →

Conus medullaris

Filum terminale

Fig. 2.33 Dorsal spine MRI: Coronal T2WI (corresponds to level 3 in Fig. 2.30)

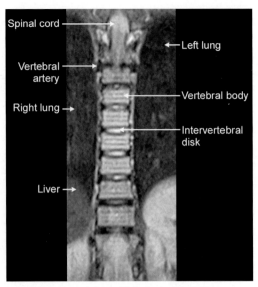

Spinal cord

Left lung

Vertebral artery

Right lung →

Vertebral body

Intervertebral disk

Liver →

Fig. 2.34 Dorsal spine MRI: Coronal T2WI (corresponds to level 4 in Fig. 2.30)

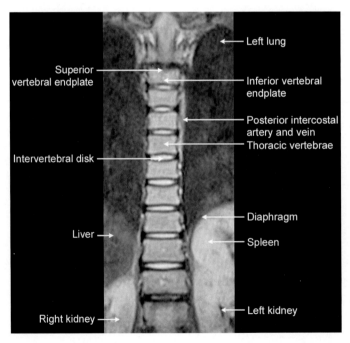

Left lung

Superior vertebral endplate

Inferior vertebral endplate

Posterior intercostal artery and vein

Thoracic vertebrae

Intervertebral disk

Diaphragm

Liver →

Spleen

Right kidney →

Left kidney

Fig. 2.35 Dorsal spine MRI: Coronal T2WI (corresponds to level 5 in Fig. 2.30)

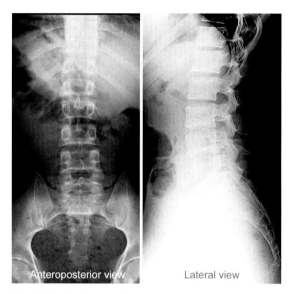

Fig. 2.36   Lumbosacral spine

Anteroposterior view

Lateral view

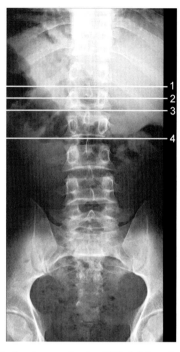

Fig. 2.37   Lumbosacral spine MRI: Axial section plan

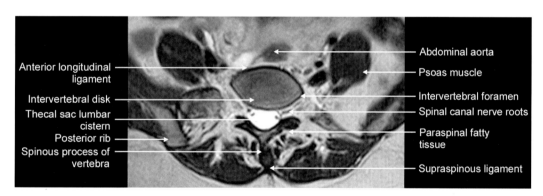

Anterior longitudinal ligament

Intervertebral disk

Thecal sac lumbar cistern

Posterior rib

Spinous process of vertebra

Abdominal aorta

Psoas muscle

Intervertebral foramen

Spinal canal nerve roots

Paraspinal fatty tissue

Supraspinous ligament

Fig. 2.38   Lumbosacral spine MRI: Axial T2WI D12-L1 disk level (corresponds to level 1 in Fig. 2.37)

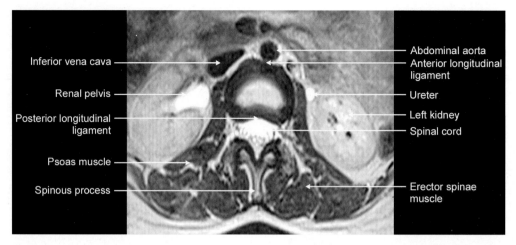

Inferior vena cava

Renal pelvis

Posterior longitudinal ligament

Psoas muscle

Spinous process

Abdominal aorta
Anterior longitudinal ligament
Ureter
Left kidney
Spinal cord

Erector spinae muscle

Fig. 2.39 Lumbosacral spine MRI: Axial T2WI L1 vertebral body level (corresponds to level 2 in Fig. 2.37)

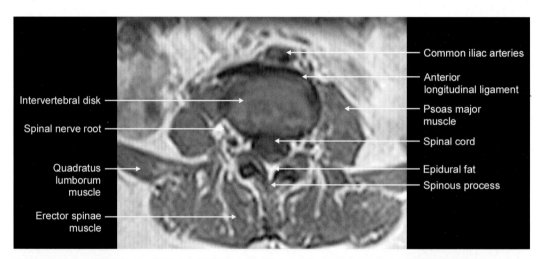

Intervertebral disk

Spinal nerve root

Quadratus lumborum muscle

Erector spinae muscle

Common iliac arteries
Anterior longitudinal ligament
Psoas major muscle
Spinal cord
Epidural fat
Spinous process

Fig. 2.40 Lumbosacral spine MRI: Axial T1WI L1-L2 disk level (corresponds to level 3 in Fig. 2.37)

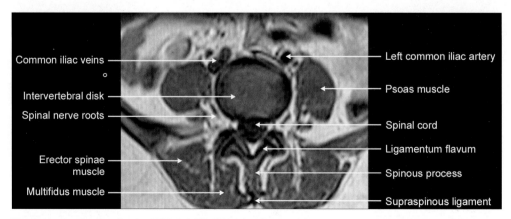

Common iliac veins

Intervertebral disk

Spinal nerve roots

Erector spinae muscle

Multifidus muscle

Left common iliac artery
Psoas muscle
Spinal cord
Ligamentum flavum
Spinous process
Supraspinous ligament

Fig. 2.41 Lumbosacral spine MRI: Axial T1WI L2-L3 disk level (corresponds to level 4 in Fig. 2.37)

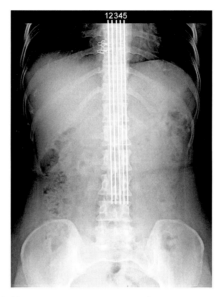

Fig. 2.42   Dorsolumbar spine MRI: Sagittal section plan

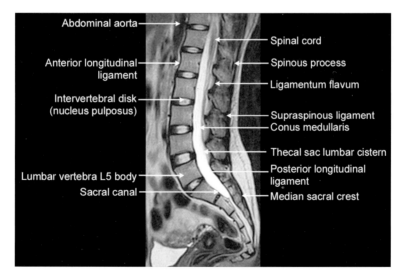

Fig. 2.43   Lumbosacral spine MRI: Sagittal T2WI (corresponds to level 1 in Fig. 2.42)

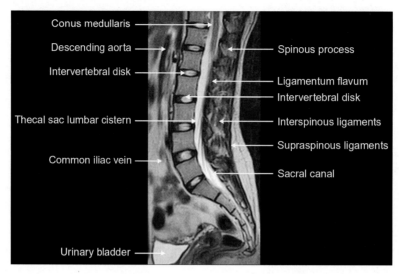

Fig. 2.44 Lumbosacral spine MRI: Sagittal T2WI (corresponds to level 2 in Fig. 2.42)

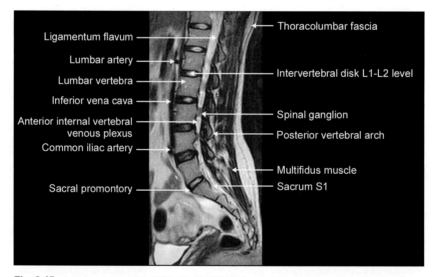

Fig. 2.45 Lumbosacral spine MRI: Sagittal T2WI (corresponds to level 3 in Fig. 2.42)

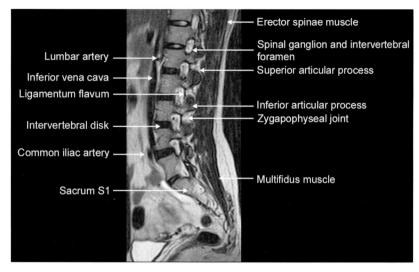

Erector spinae muscle

Spinal ganglion and intervertebral foramen

Superior articular process

Inferior articular process

Zygapophyseal joint

Multifidus muscle

Lumbar artery

Inferior vena cava

Ligamentum flavum

Intervertebral disk

Common iliac artery

Sacrum S1

Fig. 2.46 Lumbosacral spine MRI: Sagittal T2WI (corresponds to level 4 in Fig. 2.42)

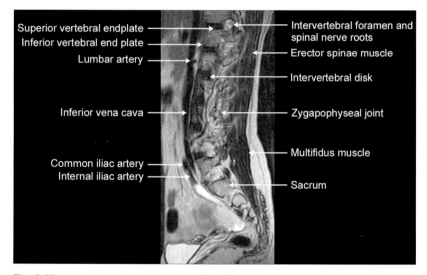

Superior vertebral endplate

Inferior vertebral end plate

Lumbar artery

Inferior vena cava

Common iliac artery

Internal iliac artery

Intervertebral foramen and spinal nerve roots

Erector spinae muscle

Intervertebral disk

Zygapophyseal joint

Multifidus muscle

Sacrum

Fig. 2.47 Lumbosacral spine MRI: Sagittal T2WI (corresponds to level 5 in Fig. 2.42)

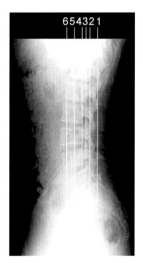

654321

Fig. 2.48 Lumbosacral spine MRI: Coronal section plan

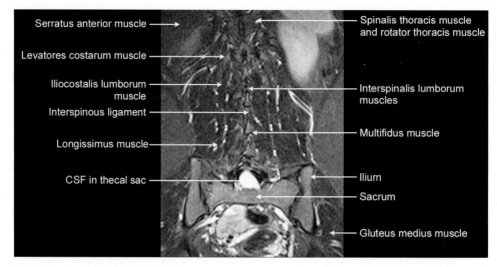

Serratus anterior muscle

Levatores costarum muscle

Iliocostalis lumborum muscle

Interspinous ligament

Longissimus muscle

CSF in thecal sac

Spinalis thoracis muscle and rotator thoracis muscle

Interspinalis lumborum muscles

Multifidus muscle

Ilium

Sacrum

Gluteus medius muscle

Fig. 2.49 Lumbosacral spine MRI: Coronal T2WI (corresponds to level 1 in Fig. 2.48)

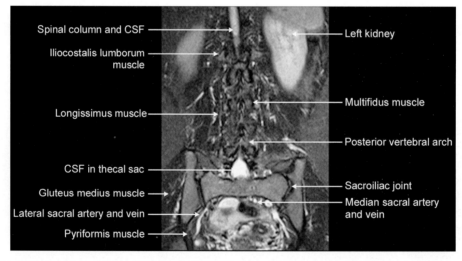

Spinal column and CSF

Iliocostalis lumborum muscle

Longissimus muscle

CSF in thecal sac

Gluteus medius muscle

Lateral sacral artery and vein

Pyriformis muscle

Left kidney

Multifidus muscle

Posterior vertebral arch

Sacroiliac joint

Median sacral artery and vein

Fig. 2.50 Lumbosacral spine MRI: Coronal T2WI (corresponds to level 2 in Fig. 2.48)

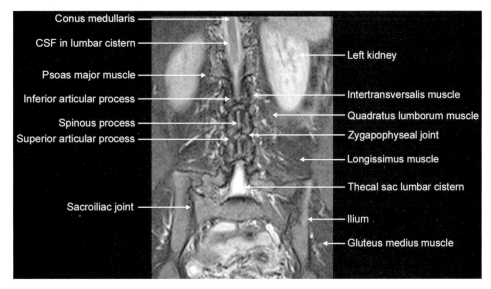

Fig. 2.51   Lumbosacral spine MRI: Coronal T2WI (corresponds to level 3 in Fig. 2.48)

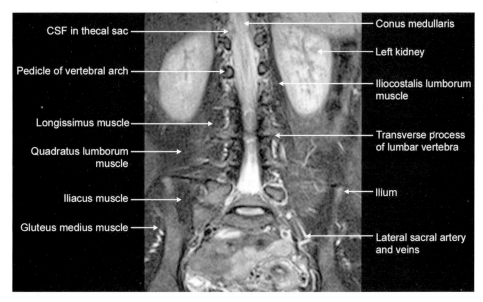

Fig. 2.52   Lumbosacral spine MRI: Coronal T2WI (corresponds to level 4 in Fig. 2.48)

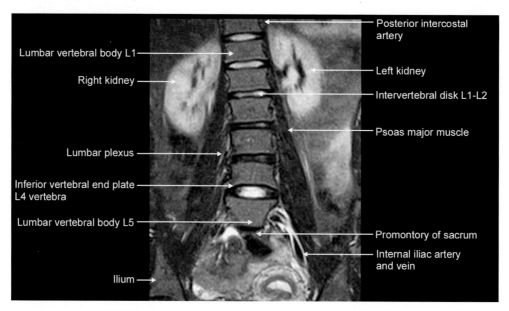

Fig. 2.53 Lumbosacral spine MRI: Coronal T2WI (corresponds to level 5 in Fig. 2.48)

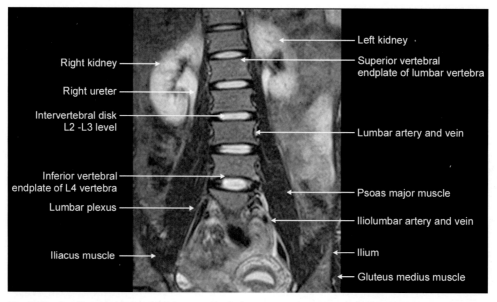

Fig. 2.54 Lumbosacral Spine MRI Coronal T2WI (corresponds to level 6 in Fig. 2.48)

CHAPTER 3

Shoulder Joint

The shoulder or glenohumeral joint is the most flexible joint in the body. It consists of bones, ligaments, muscles and their tendons, and connects the arm to the chest. It is a ball and socket joint. The glenoid cavity forms a shallow socket and is inherently unstable. The added stability to the joint is made available by the capsule, ligaments, glenoid labrum and the rotator cuff.

The articular capsule completely encircles the joint; it is attached to the circumference of the glenoid cavity beyond the labrum. Inferiorly, it is attached to the anatomical neck of the humerus.

The ligaments of the glenohumeral joint are coracohumeral ligament and glenohumeral ligaments. Glenohumeral ligament has superior middle and inferior divisions. They are designed to stabilize the shoulder in the abducted or functional position.

The labrum is a fibrocartilaginous rim attached around the margin of the glenoid cavity. It cushions and stabilizes the humerus head. It increases the superoinferior diameter of the glenoid by 75% and the anteroposterior diameter by 50%. The base of the glenoid labrum is fixed to the circumference of the cavity. It is continuous above with the tendon of the long head of the biceps, which blends with the fibrous tissue of the labrum. It deepens the articular cavity.

The tendon of the long head of biceps forms biceps-labral complex with superior glenohumeral ligament and inserts on the supraglenoid tubercle. The tendon traverses laterally in the rotator cuff interval to lie in the bicipital groove. Glenohumeral joint is in connection with the sheath of biceps tendon.

The rotator interval is the portion of the joint capsule which lies between the supraspinatus and subscapularis tendons.

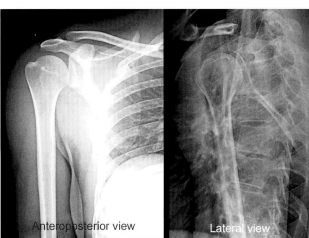

Anteroposterior view   Lateral view

Fig. 3.1 Shoulder joint

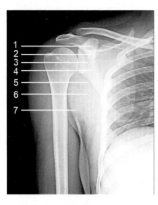

Fig. 3.2   Shoulder joint: Axial sections plan—Superior to inferior sections

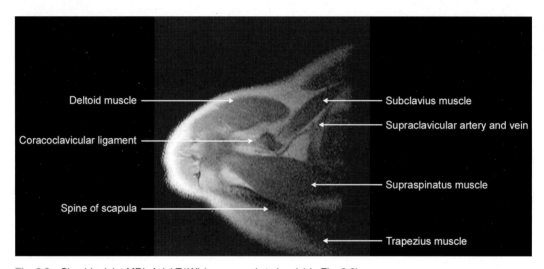

Fig. 3.3   Shoulder joint MRI: Axial T1WI (corresponds to level 1 in Fig. 3.2)

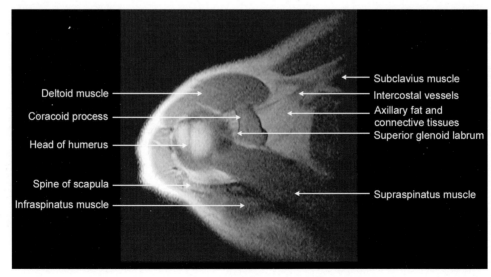

Fig. 3.4   Shoulder joint MRI: Axial T1WI (corresponds to level 2 in Fig. 3.2)

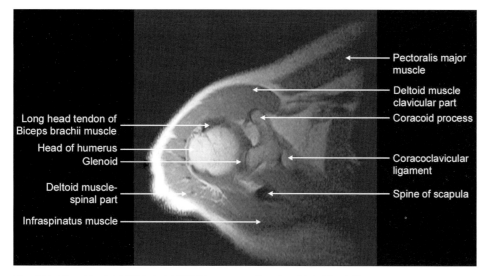

Pectoralis major muscle

Deltoid muscle clavicular part

Coracoid process

Long head tendon of Biceps brachii muscle

Head of humerus

Glenoid

Coracoclavicular ligament

Deltoid muscle-spinal part

Spine of scapula

Infraspinatus muscle

Fig. 3.5   Shoulder joint MRI: Axial T1WI (corresponds to level 3 in Fig. 3.2)

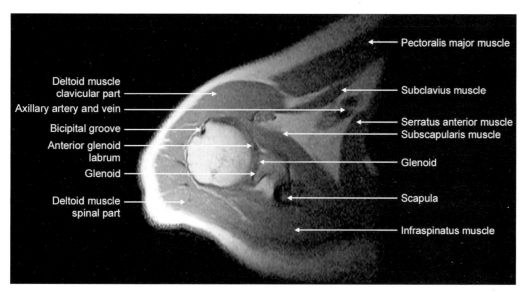

Pectoralis major muscle

Deltoid muscle clavicular part

Subclavius muscle

Axillary artery and vein

Bicipital groove

Serratus anterior muscle

Subscapularis muscle

Anterior glenoid labrum

Glenoid

Glenoid

Deltoid muscle spinal part

Scapula

Infraspinatus muscle

Fig. 3.6   Shoulder joint MRI: Axial T1WI (corresponds to level 4 in Fig. 3.2)

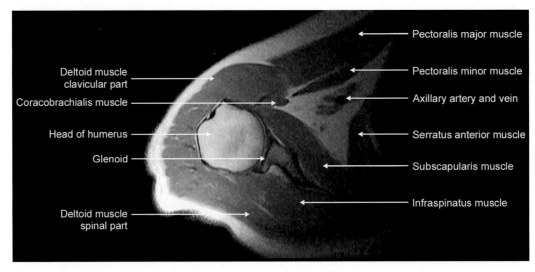

Fig. 3.7 Shoulder joint MRI: Axial T1WI (corresponds to level 5 in Fig. 3.2)

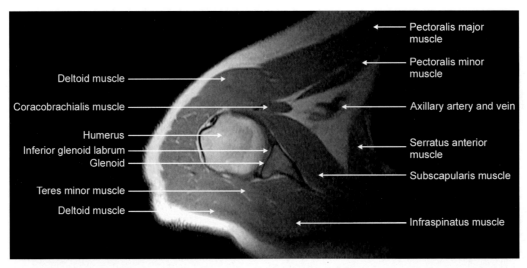

Fig. 3.8 Shoulder joint MRI: Axial T1WI (corresponds to level 6 in Fig. 3.2)

This lies between the superior and middle glenohumeral ligaments. The interval is reinforced by the coracohumeral ligament and underlying joint capsule. It is designed to limit flexion and external rotation.

Rotator cuff is formed by supraspinatus, infraspinatus, teres minor and subscapularis muscles and mostly by their flat tendons. The tendons fuse together and surround the shoulder joint. When the muscles contract, resulting in the rotator cuff tendon to rotate upward, inward, or outward. Supraspinatus tendon lies over the summit of humeral head and is an abductor. Infraspinatus and teres minor tendon cover the backside of humeral head and are external rotators. Subscapularis tendon crosses the front of the shoulder joint and is an abductot of shoulder joint.

There are two pouch-like structures the bursae located in the shoulder which produce a lubricating fluid, which helps reduce friction between the moving parts of the joint.

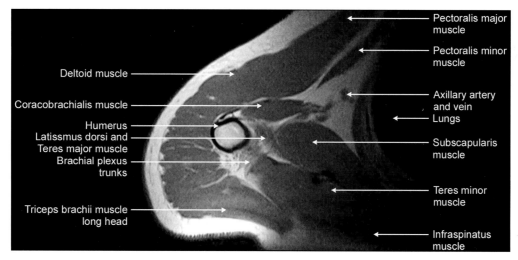

Deltoid muscle

Coracobrachialis muscle

Humerus

Latissmus dorsi and
Teres major muscle

Brachial plexus
trunks

Triceps brachii muscle
long head

Pectoralis major
muscle

Pectoralis minor
muscle

Axillary artery
and vein

Lungs

Subscapularis
muscle

Teres minor
muscle

Infraspinatus
muscle

Fig. 3.9 Shoulder joint MRI: Axial T1WI (corresponds to level 7 in Fig. 3.2)

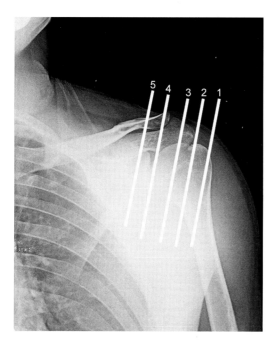

Fig. 3.10 Shoulder joint: Sagittal sections plan—Lateral to medial sections

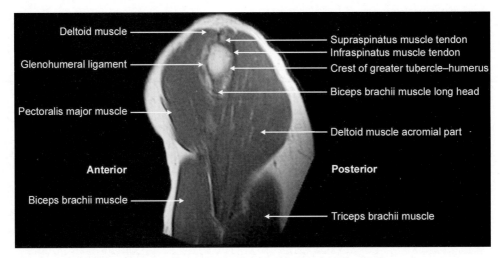

Deltoid muscle

Glenohumeral ligament

Pectoralis major muscle

Anterior

Biceps brachii muscle

Supraspinatus muscle tendon
Infraspinatus muscle tendon
Crest of greater tubercle–humerus

Biceps brachii muscle long head

Deltoid muscle acromial part

Posterior

Triceps brachii muscle

Fig. 3.11 Shoulder joint MRI: Sagittal T1WI (corresponds to level 1 in Fig. 3.10)

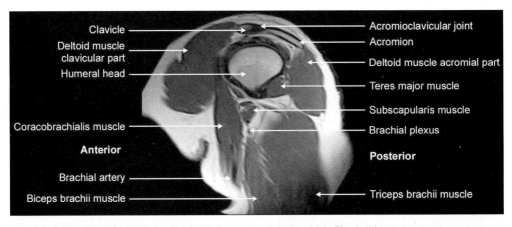

Clavicle

Deltoid muscle
clavicular part

Humeral head

Coracobrachialis muscle

Anterior

Brachial artery

Biceps brachii muscle

Acromioclavicular joint

Acromion

Deltoid muscle acromial part

Teres major muscle

Subscapularis muscle

Brachial plexus

Posterior

Triceps brachii muscle

Fig. 3.12 Shoulder joint MRI: Sagittal T1WI (corresponds to level 2 in Fig. 3.10)

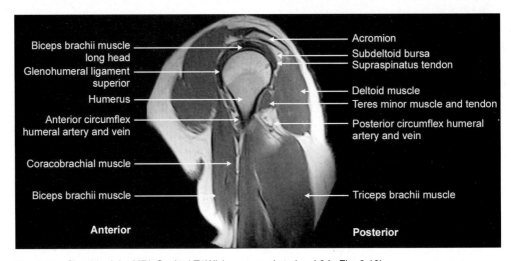

Biceps brachii muscle
long head

Glenohumeral ligament
superior

Humerus

Anterior circumflex
humeral artery and vein

Coracobrachial muscle

Biceps brachii muscle

Anterior

Acromion

Subdeltoid bursa
Supraspinatus tendon

Deltoid muscle
Teres minor muscle and tendon

Posterior circumflex humeral
artery and vein

Triceps brachii muscle

Posterior

Fig. 3.13 Shoulder joint MRI: Sagittal T1WI (corresponds to level 3 in Fig. 3.10)

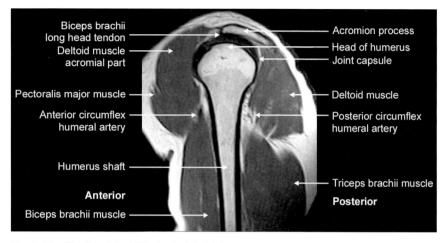

Fig. 3.14 Shoulder joint MRI: Sagittal T1WI (corresponds to level 4 in Fig. 3.10)

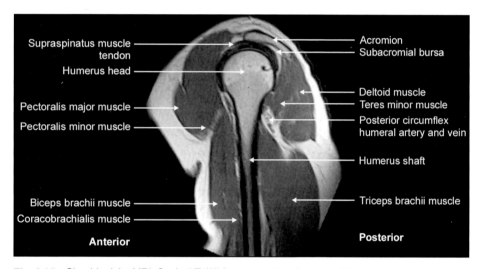

Fig. 3.15 Shoulder joint MRI: Sagittal T1WI (corresponds to level 5 in Fig. 3.10)

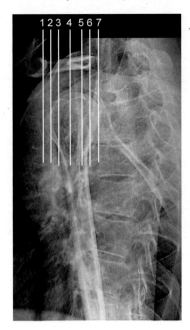

Fig. 3.16 Shoulder joint coronal sections plan

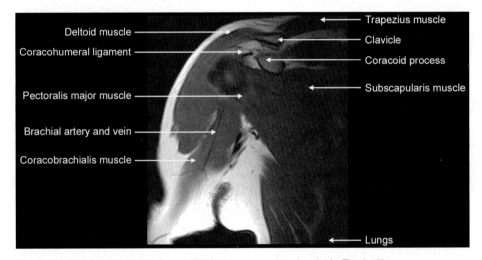

Fig. 3.17 Shoulder joint MRI: Coronal T1WI (corresponds to level 1 in Fig. 3.16)

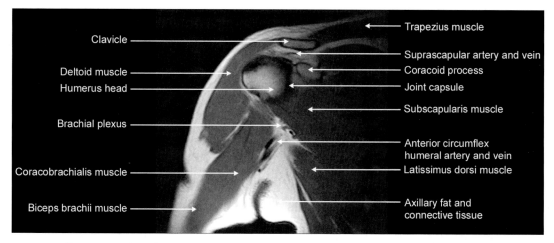

Fig. 3.18   Shoulder joint MRI: Coronal T1WI (corresponds to level 2 in Fig. 3.16)

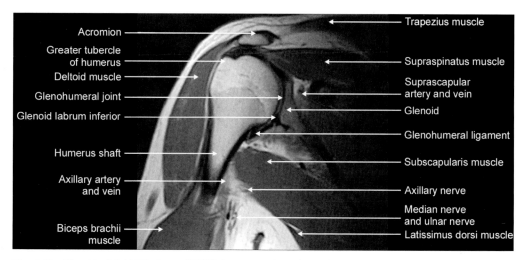

Fig. 3.19   Shoulder joint MRI: Coronal T1WI (corresponds to level 3 in Fig. 3.16)

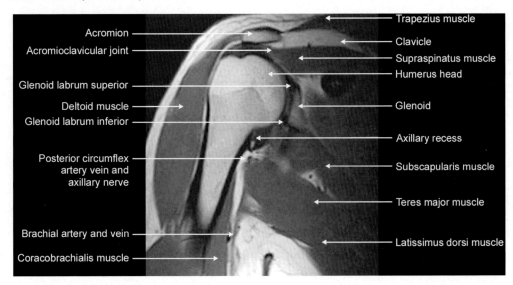

Acromion — Trapezius muscle

Acromioclavicular joint — Clavicle

Glenoid labrum superior — Suprasspinatus muscle

Deltoid muscle — Humerus head

Glenoid labrum inferior — Glenoid

Posterior circumflex artery vein and axillary nerve — Axillary recess

Subscapularis muscle

Teres major muscle

Brachial artery and vein — Latissimus dorsi muscle

Coracobrachialis muscle

Fig. 3.20 Shoulder joint MRI: Coronal T1WI (corresponds to level 4 in Fig. 3.16)

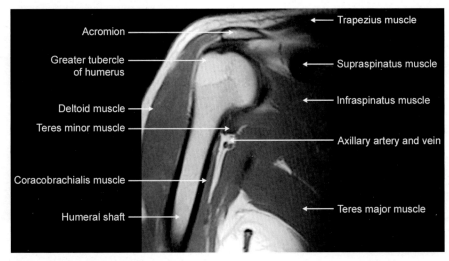

Acromion — Trapezius muscle

Greater tubercle of humerus — Suprasspinatus muscle

Deltoid muscle — Infraspinatus muscle

Teres minor muscle — Axillary artery and vein

Coracobrachialis muscle

Humeral shaft — Teres major muscle

Fig. 3.21 Shoulder joint MRI: Coronal T1WI (corresponds to level 5 in Fig. 3.16)

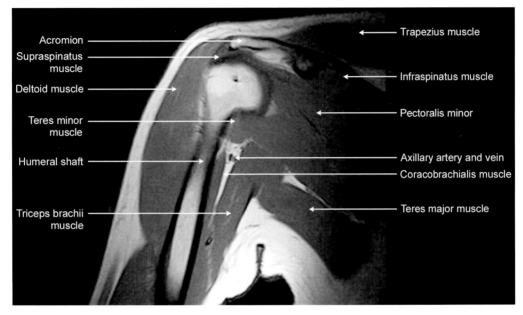

Acromion
Supraspinatus muscle
Deltoid muscle
Teres minor muscle
Humeral shaft
Triceps brachii muscle

Trapezius muscle
Infraspinatus muscle
Pectoralis minor
Axillary artery and vein
Coracobrachialis muscle
Teres major muscle

Fig. 3.22   Shoulder joint MRI: Coronal T1WI (corresponds to level 6 in Fig. 3.16)

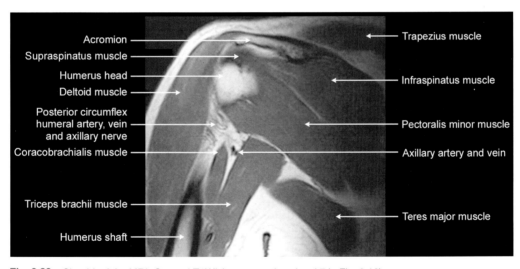

Acromion
Supraspinatus muscle
Humerus head
Deltoid muscle
Posterior circumflex humeral artery, vein and axillary nerve
Coracobrachialis muscle
Triceps brachii muscle
Humerus shaft

Trapezius muscle
Infraspinatus muscle
Pectoralis minor muscle
Axillary artery and vein
Teres major muscle

Fig. 3.23   Shoulder joint MRI: Coronal T1WI (corresponds to level 7 in Fig. 3.16)

CHAPTER 4

Upper Arm

In the arm the biceps brachii, brachialis and coracobrachialis muscles lie in the anterior compartment. The triceps brachii and anconeus muscles lie in posterior compartment. The medial intermuscular septum divides the compartments in the distal two thirds of arm. The biceps brachii muscle has two origins, the short head and the long head of the biceps. The short head of biceps originates from the tip of coracoid process of scapula, the long head orginates from the supraglenoid tubercle of scapula. The biceps brachii inserts into the tuberosity of radius and fascia of forearm through the bicipital aponeurosis. The main action of biceps brachii is to supinate the forearm. The brachialis muscle originates from the distal half of anterior surface of humerus and inserts distally into the coronoid process and tuberosity of ulna. Its action is to flex the forearm. Both the biceps brachii and brachialis muscle are innervated by the musculocutaneous nerve (C5 and C6).

The coracobrachialis muscle originates from tip of coracoid process of scapula and inserts distally into middle third of medial surface of humerus. Its action is to flex and abduct the arm. It is innervated also by musculocutaneous nerve (C5, C6, and C7).

The triceps brachii has three origins; the long head originates from infraglenoid tubercle of scapula, the lateral head from posterior surface of humerus superior to radial groove, the medial head from posterior surface inferior to radial groove. The triceps brachii inserts distally into the proximal end of olecranon of ulna and fascia of forearm. Its main action is extension of forearm. It is innervated by the radial nerve (C6, C7 and C8). The anconeus muscle arises from the lateral epicondyle of humerus and inserts distally into the lateral surface of olecranon and superior surface of ulna. Its main action is to stabilize the elbow and assist triceps brachii in extension.

The axillary artery passes inferior to the tip of coracoid process and courses posterior to the coracobrachialis . It continues as the brachial artery at the inferior border of teres major muscle. The median nerve lies adjacent to axillary and brachial arteries; it crosses the artery lateral to medial side. The ulnar nerve is adjacent to the medial side of the artery, passes posterior to the medial intermuscular septum and descends on the medial head of triceps. The musculocutaneous nerve perforates the coracobrachialis muscle and lies on the lateral side of brachial artery; it passes deeply between the biceps and brachialis muscles.

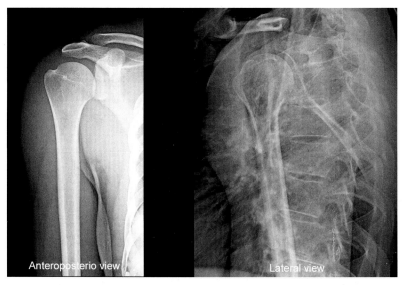

Anteroposterio view

Lateral view

Fig. 4.1 Upper arm

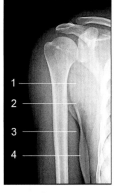

1
2
3
4

Fig. 4.2 Upper arm axial MRI: Section plan (superior to inferior sections)

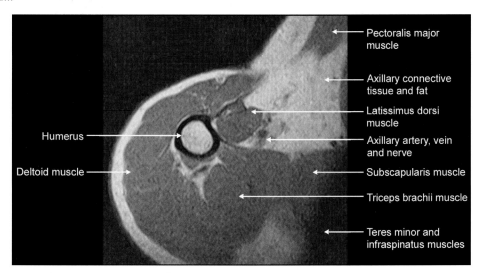

Pectoralis major muscle

Axillary connective tissue and fat

Latissimus dorsi muscle

Humerus

Axillary artery, vein and nerve

Subscapularis muscle

Deltoid muscle

Triceps brachii muscle

Teres minor and infraspinatus muscles

Fig. 4.3 Upper arm MRI: Axial T1WI (corresponds to level 1 in Fig. 4.2)

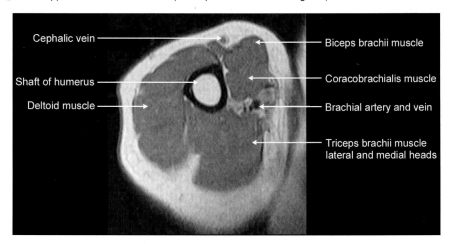

Cephalic vein

Biceps brachii muscle

Shaft of humerus

Coracobrachialis muscle

Deltoid muscle

Brachial artery and vein

Triceps brachii muscle lateral and medial heads

Fig. 4.4 Upper arm MRI: Axial T1WI (corresponds to level 2 in Fig. 4.2)

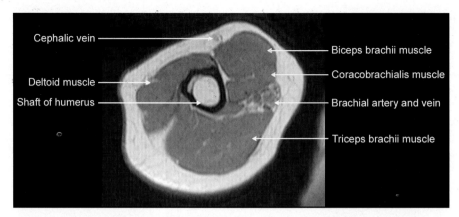

Cephalic vein

Biceps brachii muscle

Coracobrachialis muscle

Deltoid muscle

Shaft of humerus

Brachial artery and vein

Triceps brachii muscle

Fig. 4.5   Upper arm MRI: Axial T1WI (corresponds to level 3 in Fig. 4.2)

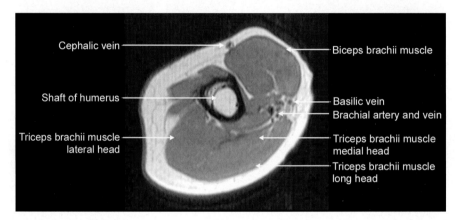

Cephalic vein

Biceps brachii muscle

Shaft of humerus

Basilic vein
Brachial artery and vein

Triceps brachii muscle
lateral head

Triceps brachii muscle
medial head

Triceps brachii muscle
long head

Fig. 4.6   Upper arm MRI: Axial T1WI (corresponds to level 4 in Fig. 4.2)

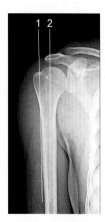

Fig. 4.7   Upper arm MRI:
Sagittal section plan (lateral
to medial sections)

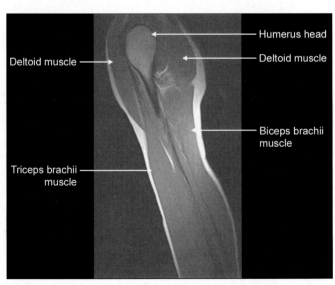

Humerus head

Deltoid muscle

Deltoid muscle

Biceps brachii
muscle

Triceps brachii
muscle

Fig. 4.8   Upper arm MRI: Sagittal T1WI (corresponds to level 1 in Fig. 4.7)

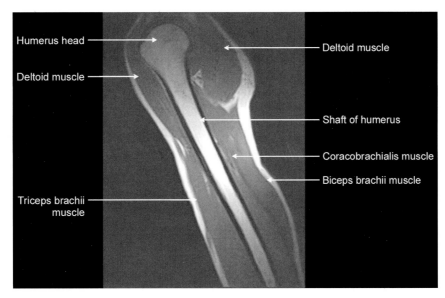

Fig. 4.9   Upper arm MRI: Sagittal T1WI (corresponds to level 2 in Fig. 4.7)

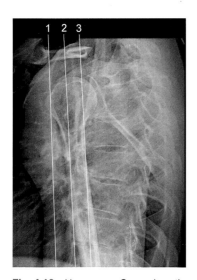

Fig. 4.10   Upper arm: Coronal section plan (anterior to posterior sections)

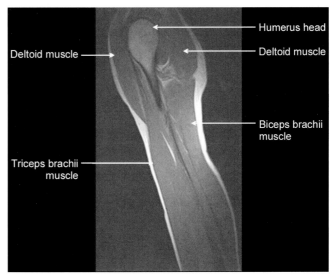

Fig. 4.11   Upper arm MRI: Sagittal T1WI (corresponds to level 1 in Fig. 4.10)

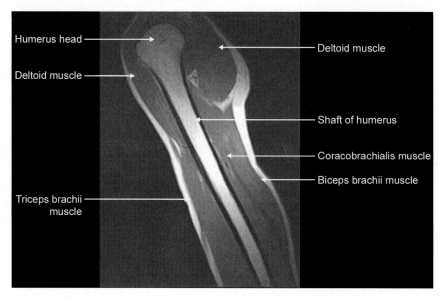

Fig. 4.12 Upper arm MRI: Sagittal T1WI (corresponds to level 2 in Fig. 4.10)

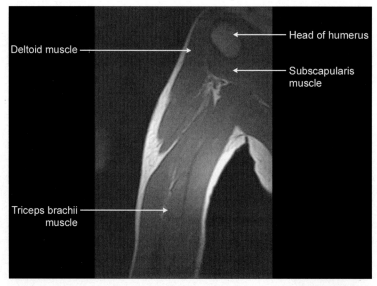

Fig. 4.13 Upper arm MRI: Coronal T1WI (corresponds to level 3 in Fig. 4.10)

CHAPTER 5

Elbow Joint

lbow joint is a hinge-type of synovial joint created by the distal humerus, proximal ulna, and radius. The distal aspect of the humerus is flat and the medial third of its articular surface, the trochlea, articulates with the ulna while the lateral capitellum articulates with the radius. On the posterior surface of the humerus is a hollow area the olecranon fossa. The posterior capsular attachment of the humerus is located above the olecranon fossa.

The anterior aspect of the distal humerus contains two fossae, the coronoid fossa, located medially, and the radial fossa, located laterally. The anterior capsular attachment to the humerus is located above these fossae.

The proximal end of the ulna has the olecranon and the coronoid process. Triceps tendon is attached to the posterior part of olecranon process. The radial head has a round shallow articular surface which articulates with the capitulum of the humerus.

A slender fibrous capsule envelops the elbow joint; a synovial membrane outlines the deep surface of this fibrous capsule. A number of fat pads are located between the fibrous capsule and the synovial membrane that is they are extrasynovial but intracapsular in position. Radial collateral ligaments and ulnar collateral ligaments reinforce the fibrous capsule.

The muscles around the elbow joint comprise of posterior, anterior, lateral, and medial groups. The muscles of the posterior group are the triceps and the anconeus. The triceps consists of three muscle bellies and attaches to the upper surface of the olecranon process of the ulna and to the antebrachial fascia

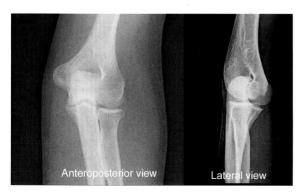

Fig. 5.1 Elbow joint

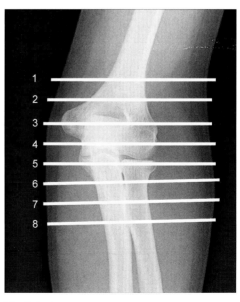

Fig. 5.2 Elbow joint axial section plan

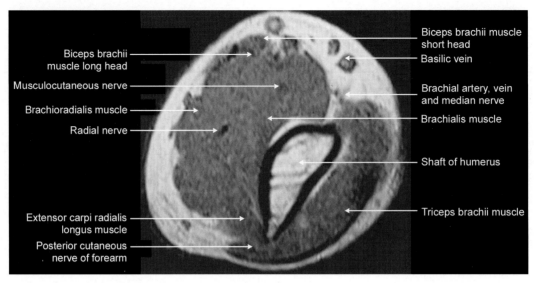

Biceps brachii muscle long head

Musculocutaneous nerve

Brachioradialis muscle

Radial nerve

Extensor carpi radialis longus muscle

Posterior cutaneous nerve of forearm

Biceps brachii muscle short head

Basilic vein

Brachial artery, vein and median nerve

Brachialis muscle

Shaft of humerus

Triceps brachii muscle

Fig. 5.3 Elbow joint MRI: Axial T1WI (corresponds to level 1 in Fig. 5.2).

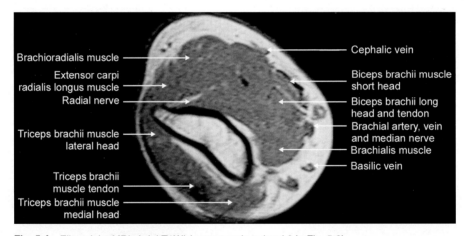

Brachioradialis muscle

Extensor carpi radialis longus muscle

Radial nerve

Triceps brachii muscle lateral head

Triceps brachii muscle tendon

Triceps brachii muscle medial head

Cephalic vein

Biceps brachii muscle short head

Biceps brachii long head and tendon

Brachial artery, vein and median nerve

Brachialis muscle

Basilic vein

Fig. 5.4 Elbow joint MRI: Axial T1WI (corresponds to level 2 in Fig. 5.2).

near the anconeus muscle. The muscles of the anterior group are the biceps and brachialis. The biceps typically consists of two heads, the short and the long head. The bellies of the biceps join to form a common tendon approximately 6-7 cm above the elbow, which attaches to the posterior aspect of the radial tuberosity. The lateral group of muscles includes the supinator and brachioradialis muscles and the extensor muscles of the wrist and hand. The medial group of muscles includes the pronator teres, the palmaris longus, and the flexors of the hand and wrist.

Brachial artery extends superficial to the brachialis muscle and medial to the biceps muscle and tendon. Three major nerves in the elbow region are median, ulnar and radial nerves. The median nerve is parallel to brachial artery and courses anterior to it in the cubital area. The ulnar nerve is present on the posteromedial part of the elbow and passes in a groove between the olecranon process of the ulna and the medial epicondyle of the humerus. The radial nerve descends and divides near the elbow into deep and superficial branches.

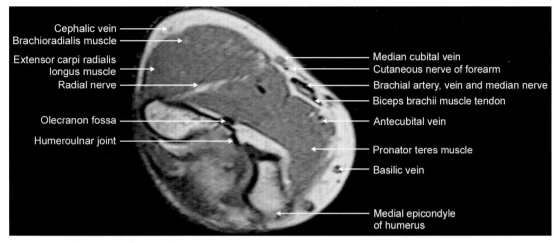

Fig. 5.5 Elbow joint MRI: Axial T1WI (corresponds to level 3 in Fig. 5.2).

- Cephalic vein
- Brachioradialis muscle
- Extensor carpi radialis longus muscle
- Radial nerve
- Olecranon fossa
- Humeroulnar joint
- Median cubital vein
- Cutaneous nerve of forearm
- Brachial artery, vein and median nerve
- Biceps brachii muscle tendon
- Antecubital vein
- Pronator teres muscle
- Basilic vein
- Medial epicondyle of humerus

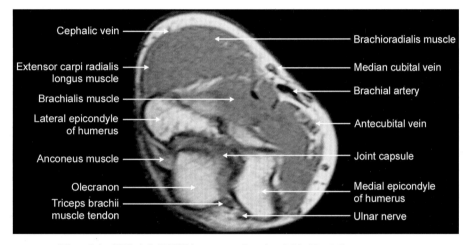

Fig. 5.6 Elbow joint MRI: Axial T1WI (corresponds to level 4 in Fig. 5.2).

- Cephalic vein
- Extensor carpi radialis longus muscle
- Brachialis muscle
- Lateral epicondyle of humerus
- Anconeus muscle
- Olecranon
- Triceps brachii muscle tendon
- Brachioradialis muscle
- Median cubital vein
- Brachial artery
- Antecubital vein
- Joint capsule
- Medial epicondyle of humerus
- Ulnar nerve

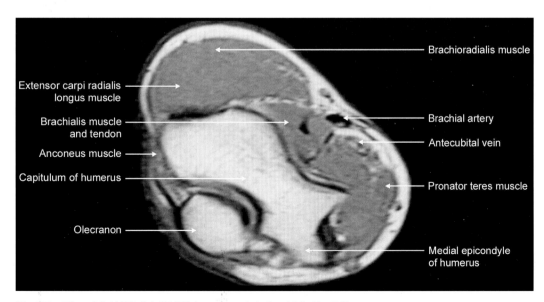

Fig. 5.7 Elbow joint MRI: Axial T1WI (corresponds to level 5 in Fig. 5.2).

- Extensor carpi radialis longus muscle
- Brachialis muscle and tendon
- Anconeus muscle
- Capitulum of humerus
- Olecranon
- Brachioradialis muscle
- Brachial artery
- Antecubital vein
- Pronator teres muscle
- Medial epicondyle of humerus

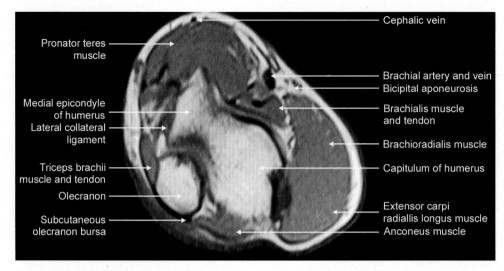

Fig. 5.8 Elbow joint MRI: Axial T1WI (corresponds to level 6 in Fig. 5.2).

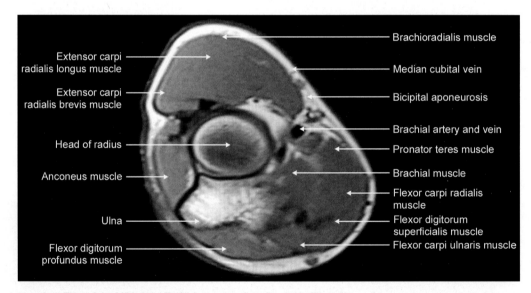

Fig. 5.9 Elbow joint MRI: Axial T1WI (corresponds to level 7 in Fig. 5.2).

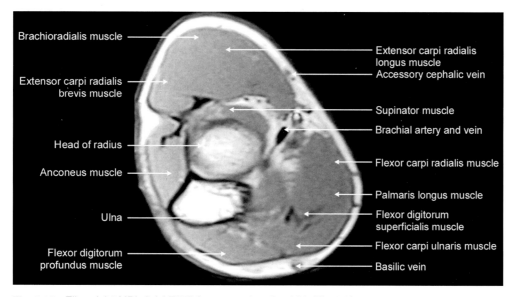

Brachioradialis muscle

Extensor carpi radialis longus muscle

Accessory cephalic vein

Extensor carpi radialis brevis muscle

Supinator muscle

Brachial artery and vein

Head of radius

Flexor carpi radialis muscle

Anconeus muscle

Palmaris longus muscle

Flexor digitorum superficialis muscle

Ulna

Flexor carpi ulnaris muscle

Flexor digitorum profundus muscle

Basilic vein

Fig. 5.10 Elbow joint MRI: Axial T1WI (corresponds to level 8 in Fig. 5.2).

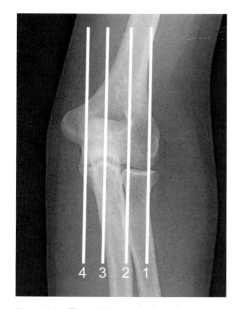

Fig. 5.11 Elbow joint sagittal section plan

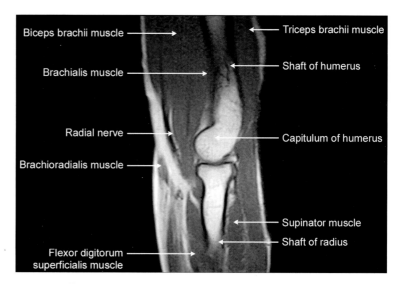

Biceps brachii muscle

Triceps brachii muscle

Brachialis muscle

Shaft of humerus

Radial nerve

Capitulum of humerus

Brachioradialis muscle

Supinator muscle

Shaft of radius

Flexor digitorum superficialis muscle

Fig. 5.12 Elbow joint MRI: Sagittal T1WI (corresponds to level 1 in Fig. 5.11).

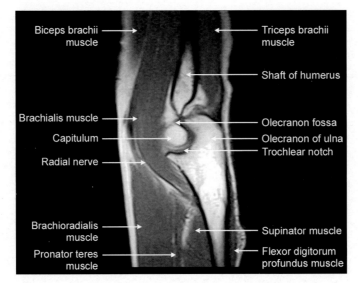

Biceps brachii muscle

Triceps brachii muscle

Shaft of humerus

Brachialis muscle

Olecranon fossa

Capitulum

Olecranon of ulna

Radial nerve

Trochlear notch

Brachioradialis muscle

Supinator muscle

Pronator teres muscle

Flexor digitorum profundus muscle

Fig. 5.13 Elbow joint MRI: Sagittal T1WI (corresponds to level 2 in Fig. 5.11).

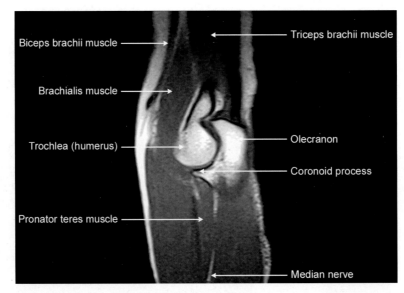

Biceps brachii muscle

Triceps brachii muscle

Brachialis muscle

Trochlea (humerus)

Olecranon

Coronoid process

Pronator teres muscle

Median nerve

Fig. 5.14 Elbow joint MRI: Sagittal T1WI (corresponds to level 3 in Fig. 5.11).

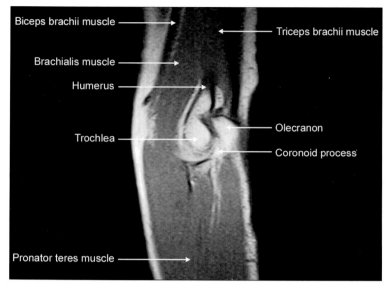

Biceps brachii muscle

Brachialis muscle

Humerus

Trochlea

Pronator teres muscle

Triceps brachii muscle

Olecranon

Coronoid process

Fig. 5.15 Elbow joint MRI: Sagittal T1WI (corresponds to level 4 in Fig. 5.11).

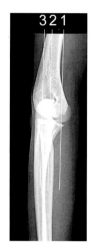

3 2 1

Fig. 5.16 Elbow joint coronal section plan

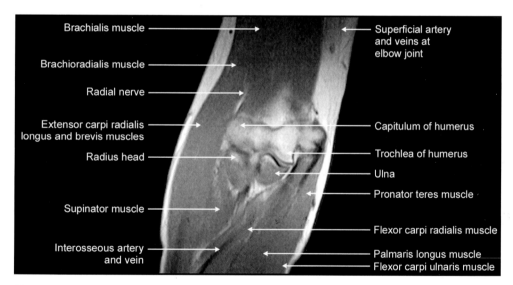

Brachialis muscle

Brachioradialis muscle

Radial nerve

Extensor carpi radialis longus and brevis muscles

Radius head

Supinator muscle

Interosseous artery and vein

Superficial artery and veins at elbow joint

Capitulum of humerus

Trochlea of humerus

Ulna

Pronator teres muscle

Flexor carpi radialis muscle

Palmaris longus muscle

Flexor carpi ulnaris muscle

Fig. 5.17 Elbow joint MRI: Coronal T1WI (corresponds to level 1 in Fig. 5.16).

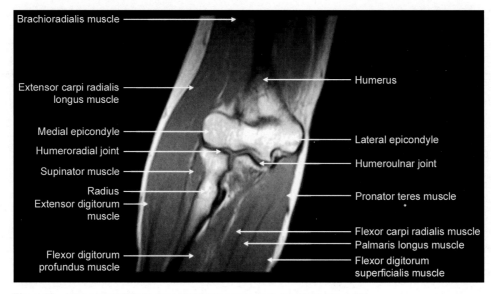

Fig. 5.18 Elbow joint MRI: Sagittal T1WI (corresponds to level 2 in Fig. 5.16).

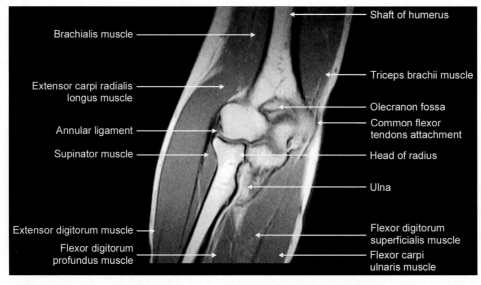

Fig. 5.19 Elbow joint MRI: Coronal T1WI (corresponds to level 3 in Fig. 5.16).

CHAPTER **6**

Forearm

The **anterior group** of muscles of the forearm are: pronator teres, flexor carpi radialis, palmaris longus, flexor carpi ulnaris, flexor digitorum superficialis, flexor digitorum profundus, flexor pollicis longus and pronator quadratus.

The **pronator teres** originates from medial epicondyle of humerus and coronoid process of ulna. It attaches distally to the lateral surface of radius. Its main action is to pronate the forearm and flex the elbow. The **flexor carpi radialis** originates from medial epicondyle of humerus and inserts distally into the base of second metacarpal. Its main action is to flex the wrist and abduct the hand. Both the pronator teres and flexor carpi radialis are innervated by median nerve (C6 and C7). The **palmaris longus** muscle arises from the medial epicondyle of humerus and inserts distally into the flexor retinaculum and palmar aponeurosis. Its main action is to flex the wrist and tightens the palmar aponeurosis. The **flexor carpi ulnaris** originates from medial epicondyle of humerus and olecranon. It inserts distally into pisiform, hook of hamate and the 5th metacarpal. Its main action is to flex the wrist and adduct the hand. The **flexor digitorum superficialis** muscle originates from the medial epicondyle of humerus and also from the superior half of anterior border of radius. It inserts distally into the middle phalanges of medial four digits. Its main action is to flex the proximal inter phalangeal joints of medial four digits and also flexes metacarpophalangeal joints. It is innervated by the median nerve (C7, C8 and T1). The **flexor digitorum profundus** originates from the medial and anterior surfaces of ulna and interosseous membrane. It inserts distally into the bases of distal phalanges of medial four digits. Its main action is to flex the distal inter phalangeal joints of medial four digits. It is innervated by both ulnar and median nerves. The **flexor**

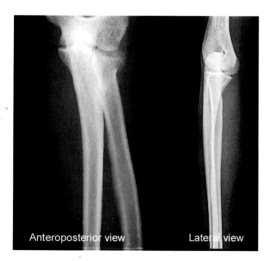

Fig. 6.1   Forearm

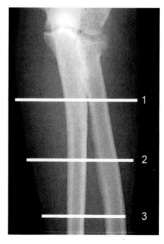

Fig. 6.2   Forearm axial section plan

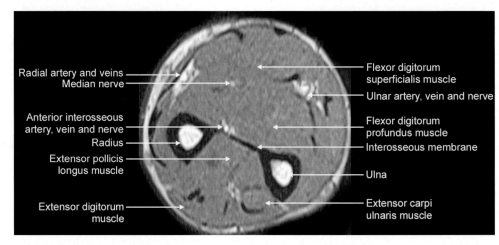

Fig. 6.3 Forearm supine MRI: Axial T1WI (corresponds to level 1 in Fig 6.2)

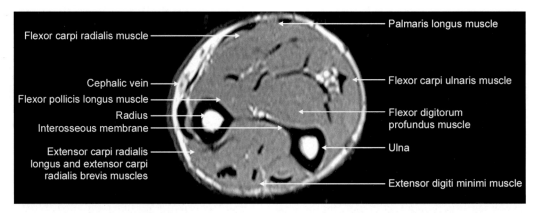

Fig. 6.4 Forearm supine MRI: Axial T1WI (corresponds to level 2 in Fig 6.2)

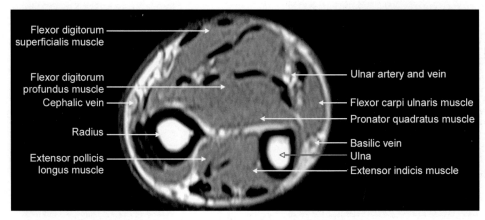

Fig. 6.5 Forearm supine MRI: Axial T1WI (corresponds to level 3 in Fig 6.2)

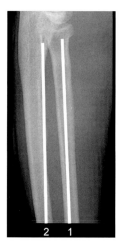

Fig. 6.6 Forearm MRI: Sagittal section plan

pollicis longus originates from anterior surface of radius and adjacent interosseous membrane. It inserts distally into the base of distal phalanx of thumb. Its main action is to flex the phalanges of first digit of thumb.

The **pronator quadratus** muscle originates from the distal fourth of anterior surface of ulna. It inserts distally into the anterior surface of radius. Its main action is pronation of forearm. Both the **flexor pollicis longus** and **pronator quadratus** mucle are innervated by anterior interosseous nerve (from median nerve (C8 and T1).

The **posterior group** of muscles of the forearm are: brachioradialis, extensor carpi radialis longus, extensor carpi radialis brevis, extensor digitorum, extensor digiti minimi, extensor carpi ulnaris, supinator, abductor pollicis longus, extensor pollicis brevis, extensor pollicis longus and extensor indicis.

The **brachioradialis** muscle arises from the upper two-thirds of the lateral supracondylar ridge, it inserts distally into the base of radial styloid. This muscle overlies the radial nerve and artery. Its main action is to flex the elbow joint. It is innervated by the radial nerve (C5 and C6). The **extensor carpi radialis longus** muscle arises from the lower third of the lateral supracondylar ridge of the humerus, it passes deep to brachioradialis and inserts distally into base of 2nd metacarpal. Its main action is extension and abduction at elbow joint. It is innervated by radial nerve (C6 and C7).

The **extensor carpi radialis brevis** muscle arises from the lateral epicondyle and inserts distally in the base of 3rd metacarpal. Its main action is extension at the wrist. It is innervated by the posterior interosseous nerve. The **extensor digitorum** muscle arises from the lateral epicondyle of humerus and divides distally into four tendons which pass under the extensor retinaculum, it inserts into the lateral four digits. Its main action is extension at the wrist. It is innervated by the posterior interosseous nerve (C7 and C8). The **extensor digiti minimi** muscle arises from the lateral epicondyle of humerus, its tendon passes under the extensor retinaculum and as it approaches the 5th digit it splits into two divisions and inserts on each side of the 5th metacarpal. Its main action is extension of the 5th digit and also assists the extensor digitorum muscle. It is innervated by posterior interosseous nerve (C7 and C8). The **extensor carpi ulnaris** muscle arises from the lateral epicondyle of humerus, distally the tendon inserts into the base of the 5th metacarpal.

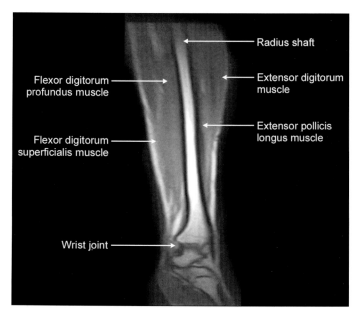

Fig. 6.7 Forearm supine MRI: Sagittal T1WI (corresponds to level 1 in Fig. 6.6)

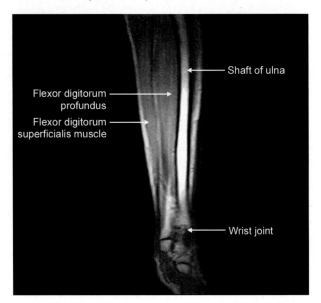

Fig. 6.8 Forearm prone MRI sagittal T1WI (corresponds to level 2 in Fig. 6.6)

Its main action is extension and adduction at the wrist. It is innervated by the posterior interosseous nerve (C7 and C8).

The **supinator** muscle arises from the distal border of lateral epicondyle and supinator crest of ulna. Its fibers run behind the radius and distally it inserts into the lateral surface of radius. Its main action is supination of forearm. It is innervated by posterior interosseous nerve (C6 and C7).

The **abductor pollicis longus** muscle arises obliquely from both bones of forearm and interosseous membrane; its ten-

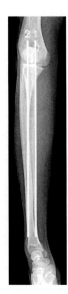

Fig. 6.9 Forearm MRI coronal section plan

don divides into two distally and attaches to the trapezium and base of first metacarpal. Its main action is extension at the first MCP joint. It is innervated by the posterior interosseous nerve (C7 and C8).

The **extensor pollicis brevis** muscle arises from the radius and interosseous membrane. It inserts distally into base of proximal phalanx. Its main action is extension at carpometacarpal and metacarpophalangeal joint of thumb. It is innervated by the posterior interosseous nerve (C7 and C8).

The **extensor pollicis longus** muscle arises from the ulna distal to abductor pollicis longus muscle. Its long tendon forms the ulnar boundary of the anatomical snuff box, it inserts distally on the dorsum of thumb. Its main action is extension of the terminal phalanx of thumb. It is innervated by the posterior interosseous nerve (C7 and C8).

The **extensor indicis** muscle arises from the ulnar surface posteriorly; its tendon remains deep and passes across the lower end of radius covered by the tendons of extensor digitorum. Its tendon inserts distally over the dorsal surface of metacarpal bone of second digit. Its main action is extension of the second digit. It is innervated by the posterior interosseous nerve (C7 and C8).

The **posterior interosseous nerve** passes through the supinator muscle fibers and enters the extensor compartment of forearm and runs closely with the interosseous membrane and innervates the muscles of extensor compartment upto the wrist joint.

The **posterior interosseous artery** passes between the forearm bones just before the interosseous membrane begins and enters the extensor compartment of forearm. It accompanies

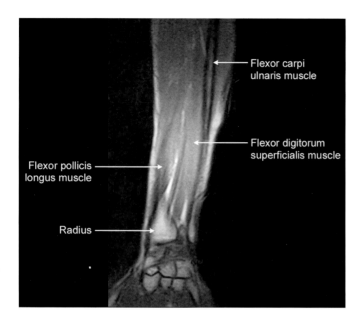

Fig. 6.10 Forearm prone MRI: Coronal T1WI (corresponds to level 1 in Fig. 6.9)

the posterior interosseous nerve and supplies the muscles of extensor compartment.

The **radial artery** passes distally medial to the biceps tendon across the supinator muscle. The brachioradialis muscle covers the muscle anteriorly in upper part of forearm. It later runs deep to the tendons of abductor pollicis longus and extensor pollicis brevis and continues as the deep palmar arch in hand.

The **ulnar artery** passes deep to pronator teres muscle, it runs close to the ulnar nerve in forearm, it passes down over the front of the wrist into the palm, where it lies in front of retinaculum and continues as the superficial palmar arch over the pisiform bone. Its main branches in forearm are the common interosseous artery which further divides into the anterior interosseous artery and posterior interosseous artery.

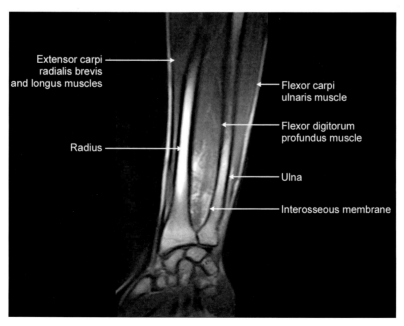

Fig. 6.11 Forearm prone MRI: Coronal T1WI (corresponds to level 2 in Fig. 6.9)

CHAPTER 7

Wrist Joint

The complex wrist joint comprises of bones and joints, ligaments and tendons, muscles and nerves. The wrist is made up of eight small carpal bones grouped in two rows. The proximal row lies where the wrist creases on bending the wrist. From lateral to medial, the proximal row of carpal bones is made up of the scaphoid, lunate, triquetrum and pisiform. The distal row is made up of the trapezium, trapezoid, capitate and hamate bones.

The distal radioulnar joint is a pivot joint formed by the head of ulna and the ulnar notch of radius, this joint is separated from the radiocarpal joint by an articular disk lying between the radius and the styloid process of ulna. The proximal radioulnar joint with the distal radioulnar joint permits pronation and supination.

In the wrist, the eight carpal bones are surrounded and supported by a watertight sac the joint capsule containing synovial fluid. It is formed by the ligaments around the wrist. The ulnar collateral ligament is on the ulnar side of the wrist and the radial collateral ligament is on the thumb side. They are two important supports on the sides of the wrist.

The distal end of ulna articulates with lunate and triquetrum. A triangular fibrocartilage complex, sits between the ulna and these carpal bones which is a small cartilage pad that cushions this part of the wrist joint. It improves the range of motion and gliding action within the wrist joint. The tendons that cross the wrist begin as muscles that start in the forearm. Those that cross the palmar side of the wrist are the flexor tendons. They run beneath the transverse carpal ligament. This band of tissue keeps the flexor tendons from bowing outward on flexion of fingers, thumb or wrist. The tendons that travel over the back of the wrist, the extensor tendons run through a series of compartments lined with tenosynovium, which prevents friction as the extensor tendons glide inside their compartment.

Three nerves that travel to the hand begin at the shoulder. The radial, the median and the ulnar nerve carry signals from the brain to the muscles that move the arm, hand, fingers, and thumb. The nerves carry back the signals to the brain about touch, pain, and temperature. The radial nerve runs along the thumb side of the forearm. It wraps around the end of the radius bone toward the back of the hand. It gives sensation to the back of the hand from the thumb to the third finger. The median nerve travels through the carpal tunnel and provides sensory function to the palmar side of the thumb, index finger, long finger and half of the ring finger. The ulnar nerve travels through the Guyon's canal formed by pisiform, hamate and the ligament that connects them and then branches to supply to the little finger and half the ring finger. Along the nerves travel the vessels that supply the hand. The radial artery runs across the front of the wrist, close to thumb. The ulnar artery runs next to the ulnar nerve through Guyon's canal. The ulnar and radial arteries arch together within the palm of the hand, supplying the front of the hand and fingers. Other arteries travel across the back of the wrist.

ERRATA

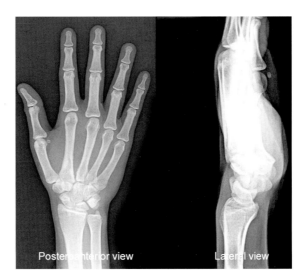

Fig. 7.1   Wrist joint

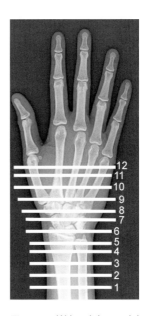

Fig. 7.2   Wrist   joint   axial section plan

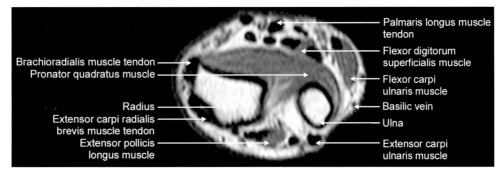

Fig. 7.3   Wrist joint MRI: Supine axial T1WI (corresponds to level 1 in Fig. 7.2)

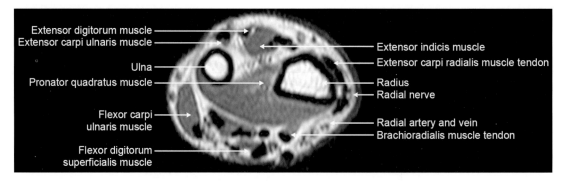

Fig. 7.4 Wrist joint MRI: Prone axial T1WI (corresponds to level 2 in Fig. 7.2)

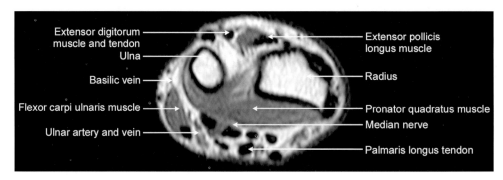

Fig. 7.5 Wrist joint MRI: Prone axial T1WI (corresponds to level 3 in Fig. 7.2)

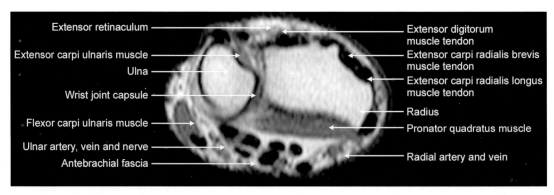

Fig. 7.6 Wrist joint MRI: Prone axial T1WI (corresponds to level 4 in Fig. 7.2)

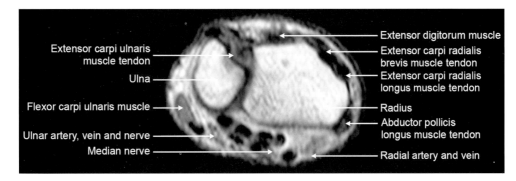

Fig. 7.7 Wrist joint MRI: Prone axial T1WI (corresponds to level 5 in Fig. 7.2)

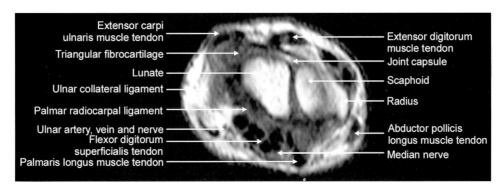

Fig. 7.8 Wrist joint MRI: Prone axial T1WI (corresponds to level 6 in Fig. 7.2)

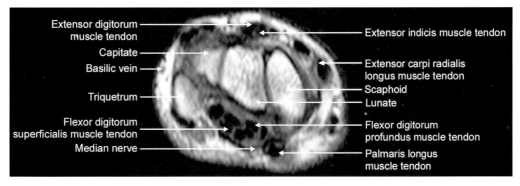

Fig. 7.9 Wrist joint MRI: Prone axial T1WI (corresponds to level 7 in Fig. 7.2)

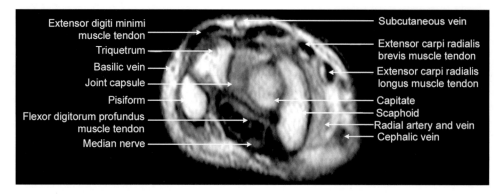

Fig. 7.10 Wrist joint MRI: Prone axial T1WI (corresponds to level 8 in Fig. 7.2)

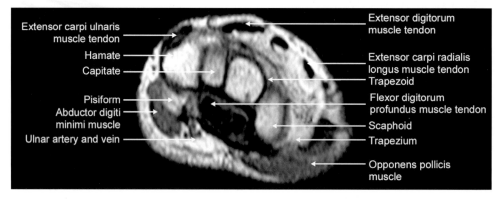

Fig. 7.11 Wrist joint MRI: Prone axial T1WI (corresponds to level 9 in Fig. 7.2)

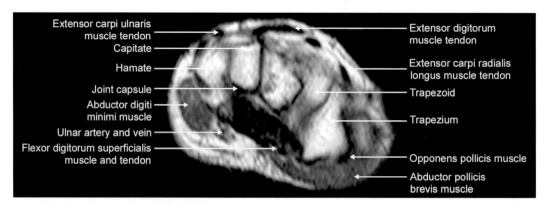

Fig. 7.12 Wrist joint MRI: Prone axial T1WI (corresponds to level 10 in Fig. 7.2)

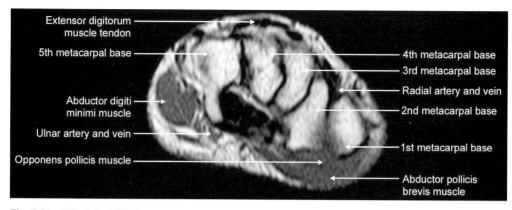

Extensor digitorum muscle tendon

5th metacarpal base

Abductor digiti minimi muscle

Ulnar artery and vein

Opponens pollicis muscle

4th metacarpal base

3rd metacarpal base

Radial artery and vein

2nd metacarpal base

1st metacarpal base

Abductor pollicis brevis muscle

Fig. 7.13 Wrist joint MRI: Prone axial T1WI (corresponds to level 11 in Fig. 7.2)

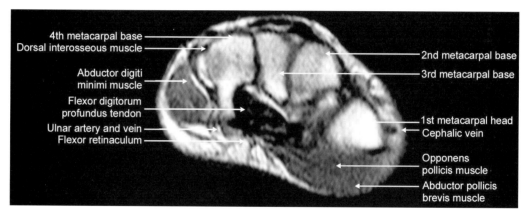

4th metacarpal base
Dorsal interosseous muscle

Abductor digiti minimi muscle

Flexor digitorum profundus tendon

Ulnar artery and vein
Flexor retinaculum

2nd metacarpal base

3rd metacarpal base

1st metacarpal head
Cephalic vein

Opponens pollicis muscle

Abductor pollicis brevis muscle

Fig. 7.14 Wrist joint MRI: Prone axial T1WI (corresponds to level 12 in Fig. 7.2)

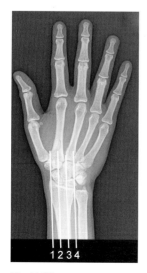

Fig. 7.15 Wrist joint sagittal section plan

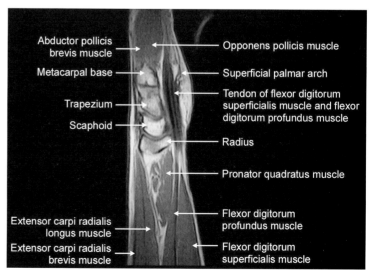

Abductor pollicis brevis muscle

Metacarpal base

Trapezium

Scaphoid

Extensor carpi radialis longus muscle

Extensor carpi radialis brevis muscle

Opponens pollicis muscle

Superficial palmar arch

Tendon of flexor digitorum superficialis muscle and flexor digitorum profundus muscle

Radius

Pronator quadratus muscle

Flexor digitorum profundus muscle

Flexor digitorum superficialis muscle

Fig. 7.16 Wrist joint MRI: Axial T1WI (corresponds to level 1 in Fig. 7.15)

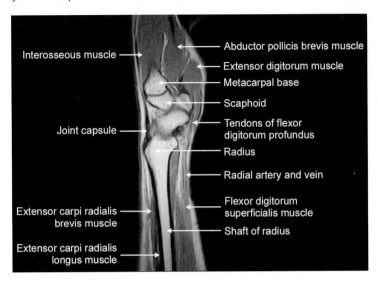

Fig. 7.17 Wrist joint MRI: Prone axial T1WI (corresponds to level 2 in Fig. 7.15)

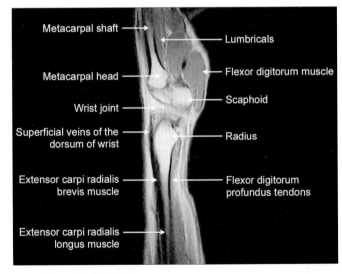

Fig. 7.18 Wrist joint MRI: Prone axial T1WI (corresponds to level 3 in Fig. 7.15)

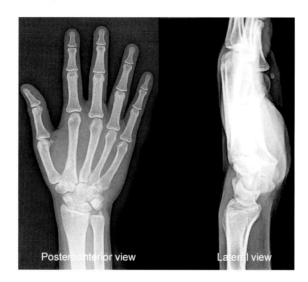

Fig. 7.1 Wrist joint

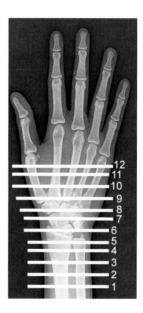

Fig. 7.2 Wrist joint axial section plan

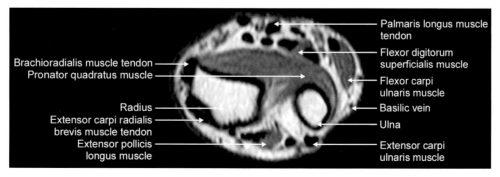

Fig. 7.3 Wrist joint MRI: Supine axial T1WI (corresponds to level 1 in Fig. 7.2)

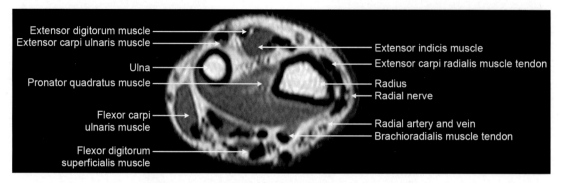

Fig. 7.4 Wrist joint MRI: Supine axial T1WI (corresponds to level 2 in Fig. 7.2)

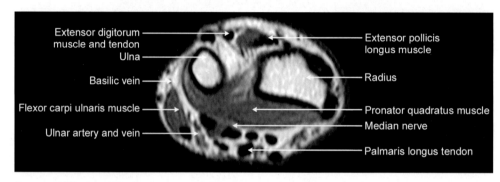

Fig. 7.5 Wrist joint MRI: Supine axial T1WI (corresponds to level 3 in Fig. 7.2)

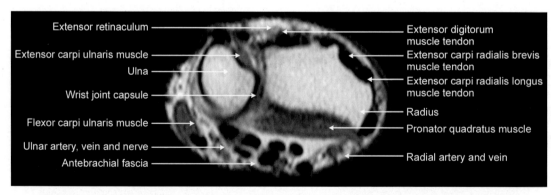

Fig. 7.6 Wrist joint MRI: Supine axial T1WI (corresponds to level 4 in Fig. 7.2)

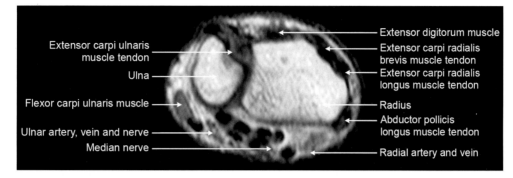

Fig. 7.7 Wrist joint MRI: Supine axial T1WI (corresponds to level 5 in Fig. 7.2)

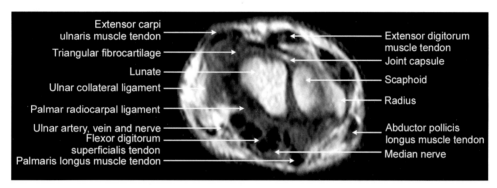

Fig. 7.8 Wrist joint MRI: Supine axial T1WI (corresponds to level 6 in Fig. 7.2)

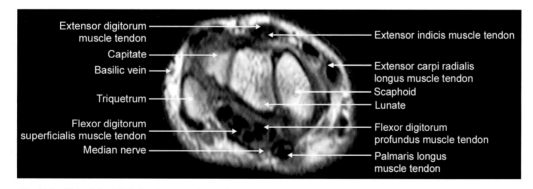

Fig. 7.9 Wrist joint MRI: Supine axial T1WI (corresponds to level 7 in Fig. 7.2)

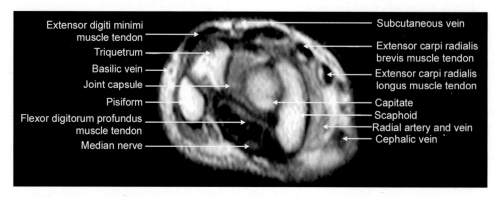

Fig. 7.10 Wrist joint MRI: Supine axial T1WI (corresponds to level 8 in Fig. 7.2)

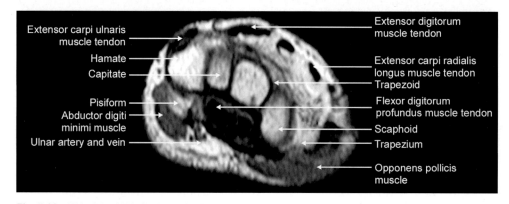

Fig. 7.11 Wrist joint MRI: Supine axial T1WI (corresponds to level 9 in Fig. 7.2)

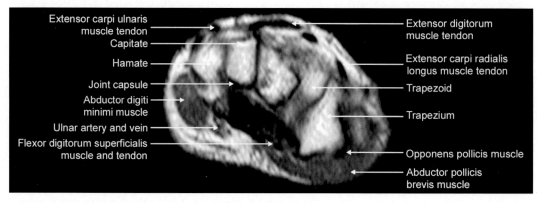

Fig. 7.12 Wrist joint MRI: Supine axial T1WI (corresponds to level 10 in Fig. 7.2)

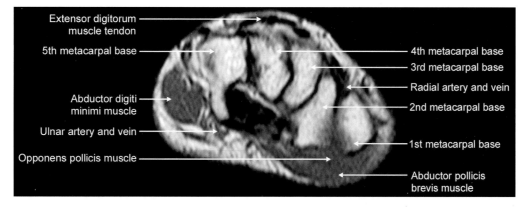

Fig. 7.13 Wrist joint MRI: Supine axial T1WI (corresponds to level 11 in Fig. 7.2)

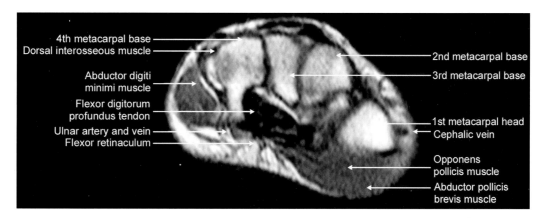

Fig. 7.14 Wrist joint MRI: Supine axial T1WI (corresponds to level 12 in Fig. 7.2)

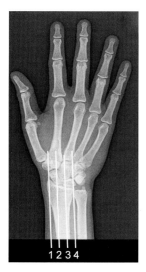

Fig. 7.15 Wrist joint sagittal section plan

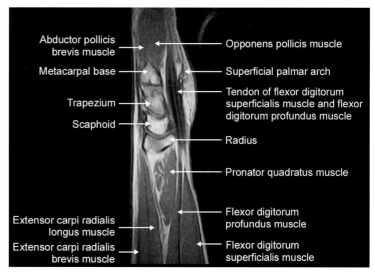

Fig. 7.16 Wrist joint MRI: Axial T1WI (corresponds to level 1 in Fig. 7.15)

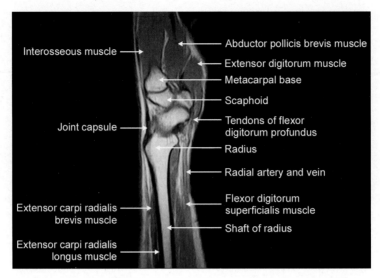

Fig. 7.17 Wrist joint MRI: Prone axial T1WI (corresponds to level 2 in Fig. 7.15)

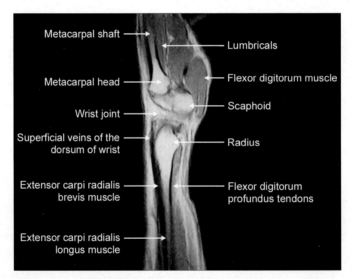

Fig. 7.18 Wrist joint MRI: Prone axial T1WI (corresponds to level 3 in Fig. 7.15)

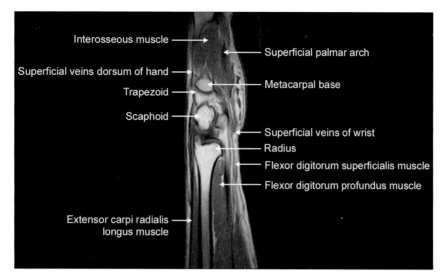

Fig. 7.19   Wrist joint MRI: Prone axial T1WI (corresponds to level 4 in Fig. 7.15)

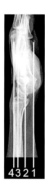

Fig. 7.20   Wrist joint MRI: Coronal section plan

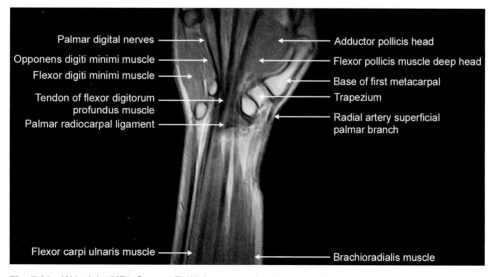

Fig. 7.21   Wrist joint MRI: Coronal T1WI (corresponds to level 1 in Fig. 7.20)

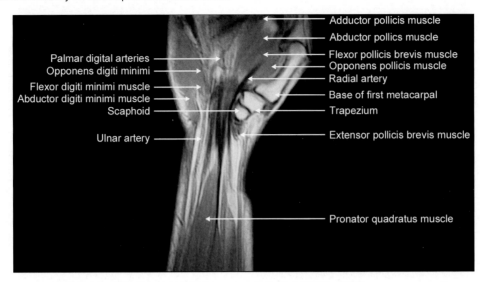

Fig. 7.22 Wrist joint MRI: Coronal T1WI (corresponds to level 2 in Fig. 7.20)

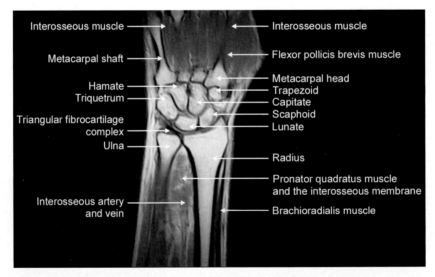

Fig. 7.23 Wrist joint MRI: Coronal T1WI (corresponds to level 3 in Fig. 7.20)

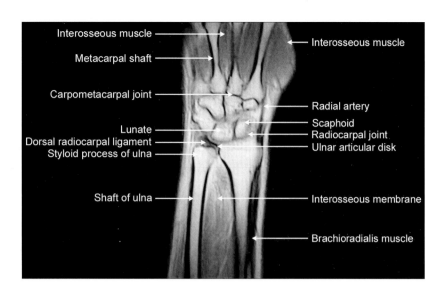

Fig. 7.24 Wrist joint MRI: Coronal T1WI (corresponds to level 4 in Fig. 7.20)

CHAPTER 8

Hip Joint

The hip joint is a multiaxial synovial joint (ball and socket joint). It engages the bony surface of the head of femur in the acetabulum of the hip bone. The stability of the joint is provided by the muscles and ligaments. The three parts of the hip bone (ilium, ischium and pubis) congregate at the acetabulum to form the triradiate synchondrosis.

The acetabular labrum is attached to the acetabular rim and the transverse acetabular ligament. It forms a complete ring encircling the head of femur which fits into the acetabular cavity. The transverse acetabular ligament bridges the acetabular notch.

At the site of the subtendinous bursa of psoas, the capsule is partially deficient and weak, is only supported by the psoas tendon. The inverted Y shaped iliofemoral ligament is attached superiorly deep to the rectus femoris muscle and becomes stiffer during medial rotation of femur at the hip joint.

The ligament of head of femur connects the head of femur to the acetabular cavity. Its fibers are also attached to the margins of acetabular notch. The ligament of the head of femur becomes stiffer during adduction movement of the hip joint, more so when the legs are crossed in front.

The fibrous capsule of the joint is strengthened by three ligaments – the iliofemoral ligament, the pubofemoral ligament and the ischiofemoral ligament. The fibrous capsule is thick where it forms the iliofemoral ligament and it is thinner posteriorly. The femoral sheath enclosing the femoral artery, vein, lymph nodes and fat is loosely bound except posteriorly between the psoas and pectinius muscles, and is attached to the capsule of hip joint. The femoral nerve lies between the iliacus muscle and the fascia. The fibers of the capsule spiral to become stiffer during movements like extension and medial rotation of the femur.

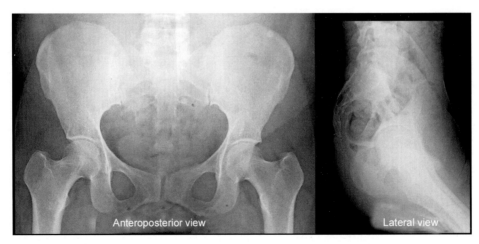

Anteroposterior view

Lateral view

Fig. 8.1 Hip joint

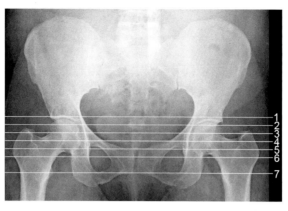

Fig. 8.2   Hip joint axial section plan

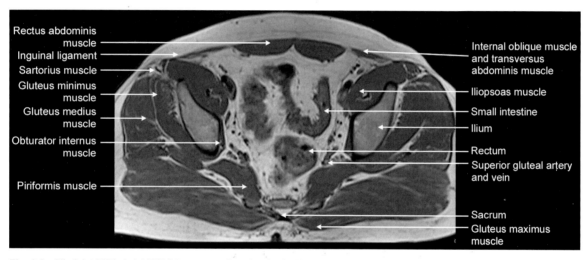

Fig. 8.3   Hip joint MRI: Axial T1WI (corresponds to level 1 in Fig. 8.2)

The synovial membrane inferiorly forms a bursa for the tendon of obturator externus muscle. The subtendinous bursa of the obturator internus is seen at the lesser sciatic notch, where the tendon makes an angle of 90⁰ to attach to the greater trochanter.

The obturator artery divides into anterior and posterior branches. The acetabular artery is a branch of the posterior branch of obturator artery. The acetabular branches pass through the acetabular foramen and enter the acetabular fossa where they diverge in the fatty tissue. The nutrient branches radiate to the margins of the acetabular fossa to enter the nutrient foramina. Major anastomosis occurs around the femoral neck involving branches from the femoral arteries (medial and lateral circumflex branches) and obturator artery branches. As the medial circumflex artery supplies a major portion of blood to the head and neck of femur, in fracture of femoral neck this blood supply is disrupted and the head of femur may undergo avascular necrosis.

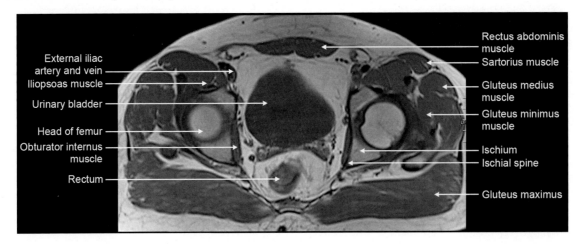

Fig. 8.4 Hip joint MRI: Axial T1WI (corresponds to level 2 in Fig. 8.2)

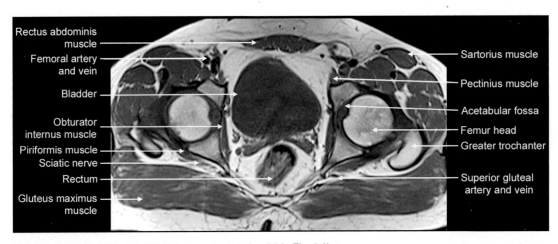

Fig. 8.5 Hip joint MRI: Axial T1WI (corresponds to level 3 in Fig. 8.2)

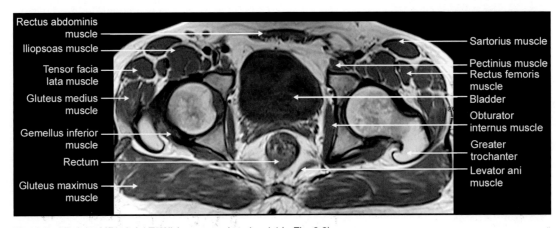

Fig. 8.6 Hip joint MRI: Axial T1WI (corresponds to level 4 in Fig. 8.2)

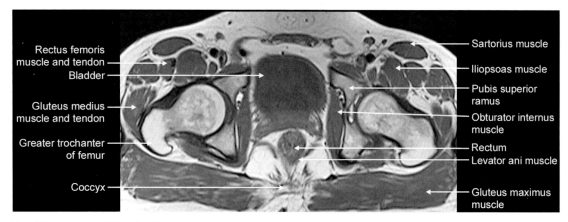

Rectus femoris muscle and tendon
Bladder
Gluteus medius muscle and tendon
Greater trochanter of femur
Coccyx

Sartorius muscle
Iliopsoas muscle
Pubis superior ramus
Obturator internus muscle
Rectum
Levator ani muscle
Gluteus maximus muscle

Fig. 8.7 Hip joint MRI: Axial T1WI (corresponds to level 5 in Fig. 8.2)

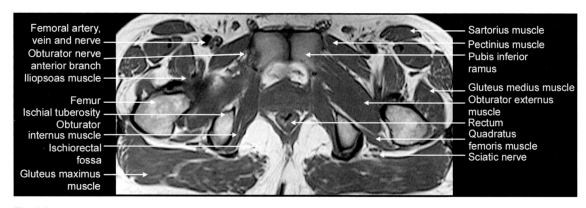

Femoral artery, vein and nerve
Obturator nerve anterior branch
Iliopsoas muscle
Femur
Ischial tuberosity
Obturator internus muscle
Ischiorectal fossa
Gluteus maximus muscle

Sartorius muscle
Pectinius muscle
Pubis inferior ramus
Gluteus medius muscle
Obturator externus muscle
Rectum
Quadratus femoris muscle
Sciatic nerve

Fig. 8.8 Hip joint MRI: Axial T1WI (corresponds to level 6 in Fig. 8.2)

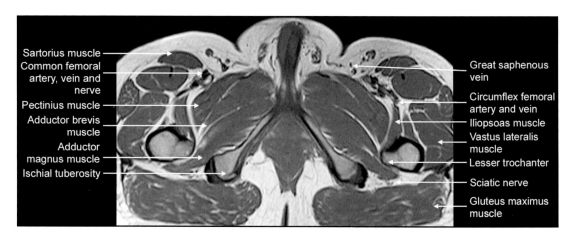

Sartorius muscle
Common femoral artery, vein and nerve
Pectinius muscle
Adductor brevis muscle
Adductor magnus muscle
Ischial tuberosity

Great saphenous vein
Circumflex femoral artery and vein
Iliopsoas muscle
Vastus lateralis muscle
Lesser trochanter
Sciatic nerve
Gluteus maximus muscle

Fig. 8.9 Hip joint MRI: Axial T1WI (corresponds to level 7 in Fig. 8.2)

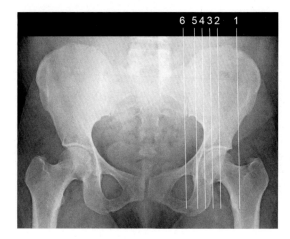

Fig. 8.10 Hip joint sagittal section plan

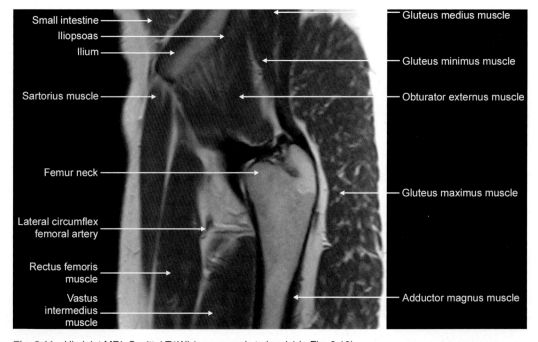

Fig. 8.11 Hip joint MRI: Sagittal T1WI (corresponds to level 1 in Fig. 8.10)

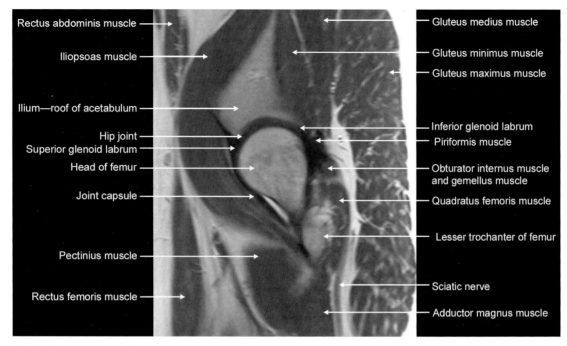

Rectus abdominis muscle

Iliopsoas muscle

Ilium—roof of acetabulum

Hip joint
Superior glenoid labrum
Head of femur

Joint capsule

Pectinius muscle

Rectus femoris muscle

Gluteus medius muscle

Gluteus minimus muscle
Gluteus maximus muscle

Inferior glenoid labrum
Piriformis muscle
Obturator internus muscle
and gemellus muscle
Quadratus femoris muscle

Lesser trochanter of femur

Sciatic nerve

Adductor magnus muscle

Fig. 8.12   Hip joint MRI: Sagittal T1WI (corresponds to level 2 in Fig. 8.10)

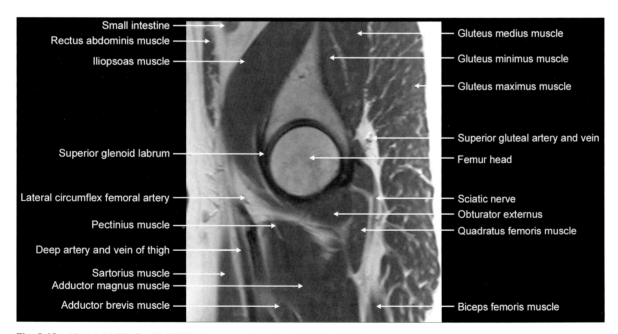

Small intestine
Rectus abdominis muscle
Iliopsoas muscle

Superior glenoid labrum

Lateral circumflex femoral artery

Pectinius muscle

Deep artery and vein of thigh

Sartorius muscle
Adductor magnus muscle
Adductor brevis muscle

Gluteus medius muscle

Gluteus minimus muscle

Gluteus maximus muscle

Superior gluteal artery and vein
Femur head

Sciatic nerve
Obturator externus
Quadratus femoris muscle

Biceps femoris muscle

Fig. 8.13   Hip joint MRI: Sagittal T1WI (corresponds to level 3 in Fig. 8.10)

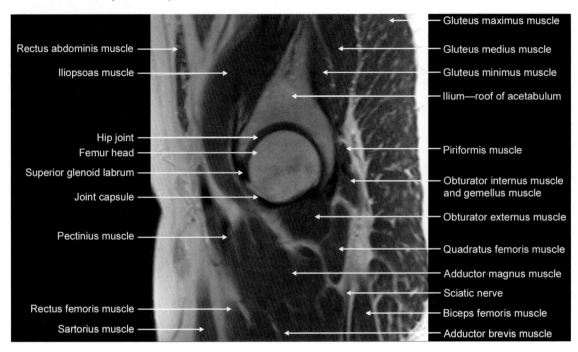

Fig. 8.14 Hip joint MRI: Sagittal T1WI (corresponds to level 4 in Fig. 8.10)

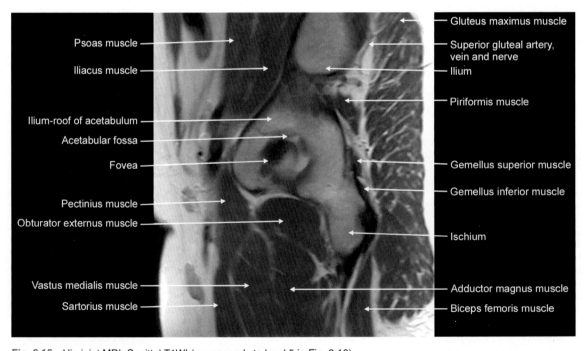

Fig. 8.15 Hip joint MRI: Sagittal T1WI (corresponds to level 5 in Fig. 8.10)

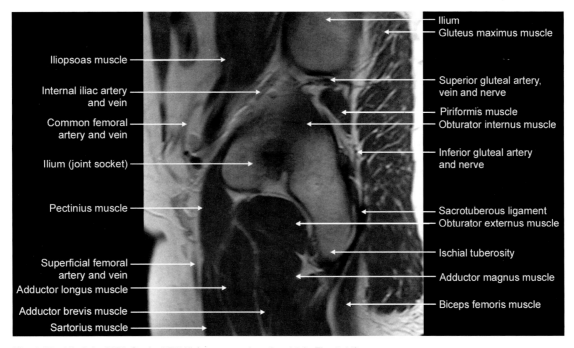

Iliopsoas muscle

Internal iliac artery and vein

Common femoral artery and vein

Ilium (joint socket)

Pectinius muscle

Superficial femoral artery and vein

Adductor longus muscle

Adductor brevis muscle

Sartorius muscle

Ilium

Gluteus maximus muscle

Superior gluteal artery, vein and nerve

Piriformis muscle

Obturator internus muscle

Inferior gluteal artery and nerve

Sacrotuberous ligament

Obturator externus muscle

Ischial tuberosity

Adductor magnus muscle

Biceps femoris muscle

Fig. 8.16 Hip joint MRI: Sagittal T1WI (corresponds to level 6 in Fig. 8.10)

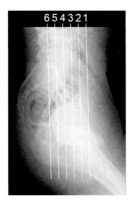

Fig. 8.17 Hip joint coronal section plan

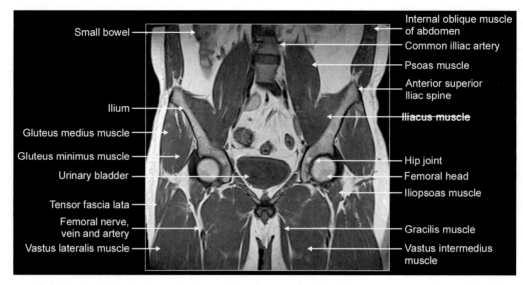

Fig. 8.18 Hip joint MRI: Coronal T1WI (corresponds to level 1 in Fig. 8.17)

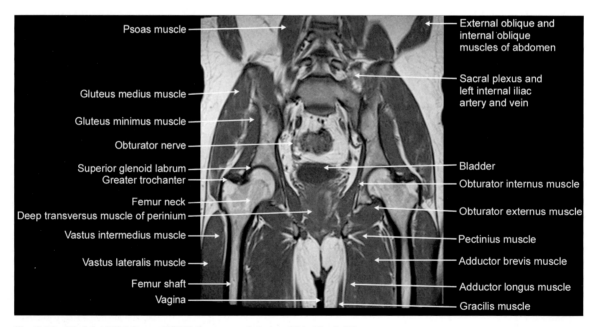

Fig. 8.19 Hip joint MR:I Coronal T1WI (corresponds to level 2 in Fig. 8.17)

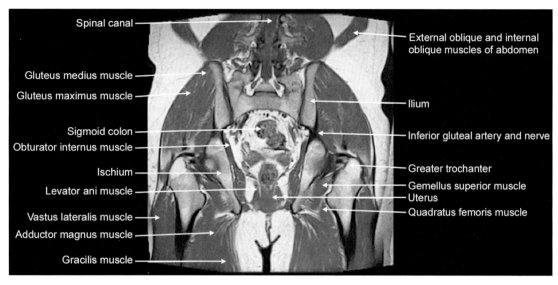

Fig. 8.20   Hip joint MRI: Coronal T1WI (corresponds to level 3 in Fig. 8.17)

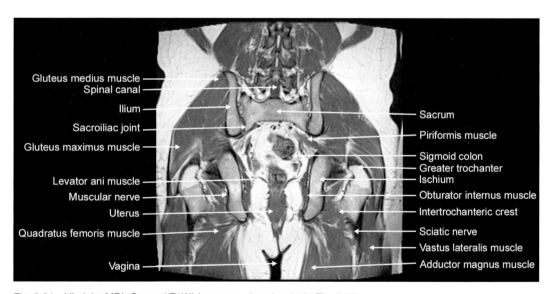

Fig. 8.21   Hip joint MRI: Coronal T1WI (corresponds to level 4 in Fig. 8.17)

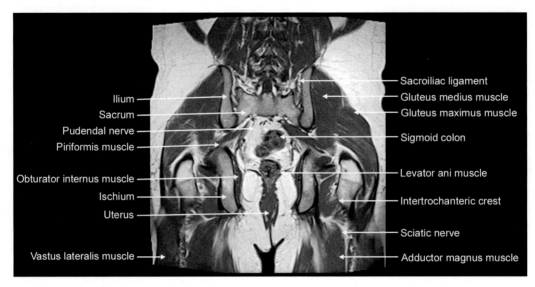

Ilium
Sacrum
Pudendal nerve
Piriformis muscle
Obturator internus muscle
Ischium
Uterus
Vastus lateralis muscle

Sacroiliac ligament
Gluteus medius muscle
Gluteus maximus muscle
Sigmoid colon
Levator ani muscle
Intertrochanteric crest
Sciatic nerve
Adductor magnus muscle

Fig. 8.22 Hip joint MRI: Coronal T1WI (corresponds to level 5 in Fig. 8.17)

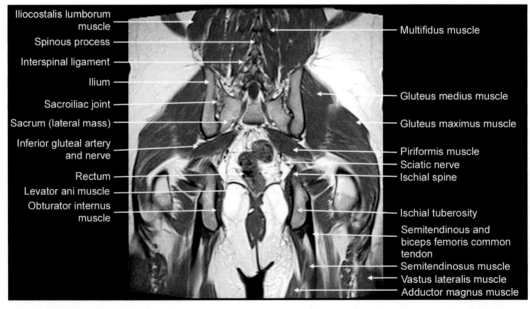

Iliocostalis lumborum muscle
Spinous process
Interspinal ligament
Ilium
Sacroiliac joint
Sacrum (lateral mass)
Inferior gluteal artery and nerve
Rectum
Levator ani muscle
Obturator internus muscle

Multifidus muscle
Gluteus medius muscle
Gluteus maximus muscle
Piriformis muscle
Sciatic nerve
Ischial spine
Ischial tuberosity
Semitendinous and biceps femoris common tendon
Semitendinosus muscle
Vastus lateralis muscle
Adductor magnus muscle

Fig. 8.23 Hip joint MRI: Coronal T1WI (corresponds to level 6 in Fig. 8.17)

CHAPTER **9**

Thigh

The muscle groups of the thigh provide support to the hip and knee joints and help in movement. The main muscle groups are – the anterior, medial, gluteal region, posterior thigh muscles and iliotibial tract on lateral aspect.

The muscles of the anterior thigh are the iliopsoas and quadriceps femoris. The iliopsoas muscle group consists of the psoas major, iliacus, tensor fascia lata and sartorius. The iliopsoas muscles are attached to the transverse process of all lumbar vertebrae, iliac crest and sacroiliac joints. The ilio-

psoas muscle is distally attached to the lesser trochanter of femur. The tensor fascia lata is attached cranially to the antero-superior iliac spine and distally it is attached to the lateral condyle of tibia. The sartorius muscle is superiorly attached to the anterosuperior iliac spine and distally inserted to the superior surface of medial surface of tibia. These muscles are supplied by L1, L2, L3 nerves and superior gluteal nerve. The main action of this group of muscles at the hip is flexion and medial rotation movements.

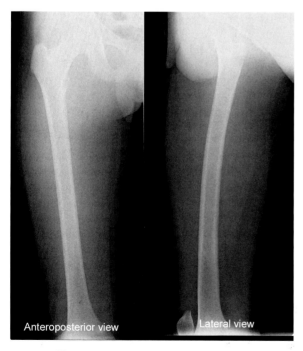

Fig. 9.1   Thigh

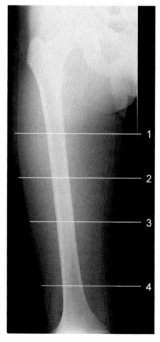

Fig. 9.2   Thigh axial section plan

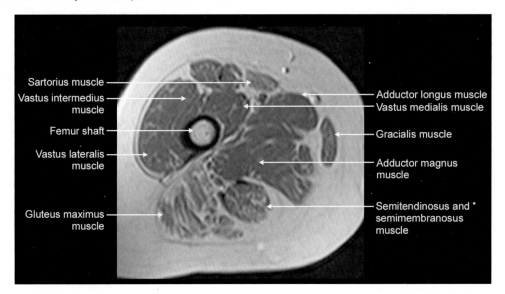

Sartorius muscle

Vastus intermedius muscle

Femur shaft

Vastus lateralis muscle

Gluteus maximus muscle

Adductor longus muscle

Vastus medialis muscle

Gracialis muscle

Adductor magnus muscle

Semitendinosus and semimembranosus muscle

Fig. 9.3 Thigh MRI: Axial T1WI (corresponds to level 1 in Fig. 9.2)

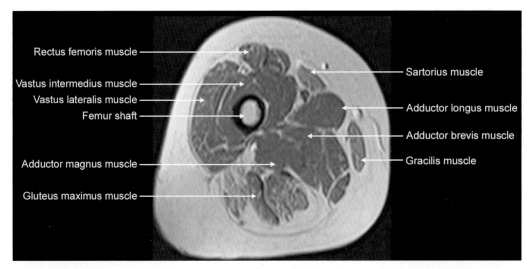

Rectus femoris muscle

Vastus intermedius muscle

Vastus lateralis muscle

Femur shaft

Adductor magnus muscle

Gluteus maximus muscle

Sartorius muscle

Adductor longus muscle

Adductor brevis muscle

Gracilis muscle

Fig. 9.4 Thigh MRI: Axial T1WI (corresponds to level 2 in Fig. 9.2)

The quadriceps femoris muscle group consists of four muscles: the rectus femoris, vastus lateralis, vastus medialis and vastus intermedius muscles. The quadriceps group of tendons congregate inferiorly to fuse together and attach to the base of the patella. The patella in turn through the patellar tendon is attached to the tibial tuberosity. Quadriceps muscles are innervated by the femoral nerve (L2 to L4). The main action of these muscles is extension at knee joint.

The muscle of the medial aspect of thigh are: the pectineus, adductor longus, adductor brevis, adductor magnus, gracilis and obturator externus muscles. The adductor group of muscles arise from the pubic bone and insert inferiorly and medially into the pectineal line and linea aspera of proximal femur. Gracilis muscle arises from the pubic ramus and inserts distally into the trochanteric fossa of femur. These muscles are innervated by L2, L3, L4 nerves. The action at the hip is adduction and flexion movements.

The muscles of the gluteal region are: gluteus maximus, gluteus medius, gluteus minimus, pyriformis, obturator internus, gemelli (superior and inferior), quadratus femoris. These gluteal muscles are attached to the dorsal surface of sacrum and ilium. They are attached inferiorly to the greater

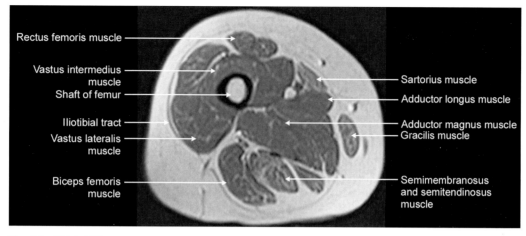

Fig. 9.5 Thigh MRI: Axial T1WI (corresponds to level 3 in Fig. 9.2)

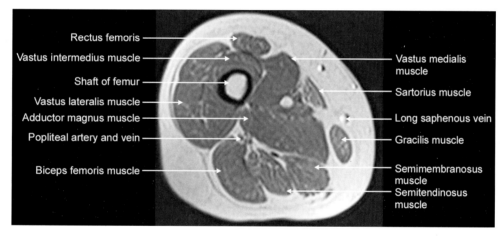

Fig. 9.6 Thigh MRI: Axial T1WI (corresponds to level 4 in Fig. 9.2)

trochanter and the intertrochanteric crest of femur. They perform extension, abduction, medial and lateral rotation at the thigh. These muscles are innervated by L5, S1 and S2 nerves.

The muscles of the posterior thigh are hamstring muscles, namely: semitendinosus, semimembranosus and biceps femoris muscles. The semitendinosus and semimembranosus muscles have a common origin from the ischial tuberosity and are attached inferiorly to the medial condyle and surface of tibia. Their main action is extension, flexion and medial rotation of the leg. These muscles are innervated by tibial division of sciatic nerve (L5, S1 and S2). The long head of biceps femoris originates from the ischial tuberosity, the short

head from supracondylar line of femur and inserts into the lateral side of head of fibula. The tendon of biceps femoris is split inferiorly by the fibular collateral ligament of knee. Its main action is in flexion and lateral rotation of leg, and extension of the thigh.

The posterior edge of the iliotibial tract serves as a tendon for the gluteus maximus and tensor fascia lata. It attaches to the lateral condyle of tibia and stabilizes the hip and knee joints during extension and flexion movements.

The sciatic nerve runs vertically downward through the hamstring compartment, lying deep to the long head of biceps femoris and adductor magnus muscles, at the apex of the popliteal fossa it divides into its tibial and common peroneal branches.

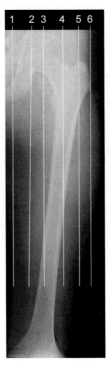

Fig. 9.7   Thigh sagittal section plan

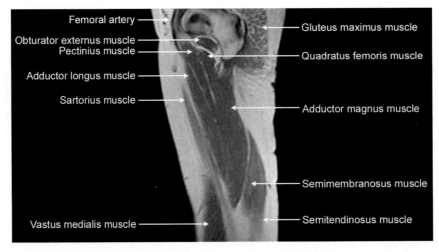

Fig. 9.8   Thigh MRI: Sagittal T1WI (corresponds to level 1 in Fig. 9.7)

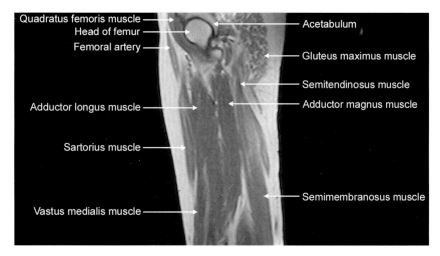

Fig. 9.9 Thigh MRI: Sagittal T1WI (corresponds to level 2 in Fig. 9.7)

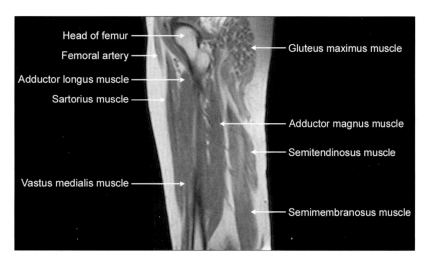

Fig. 9.10 Thigh MRI: Sagittal T1WI (corresponds to level 3 in Fig. 9.7)

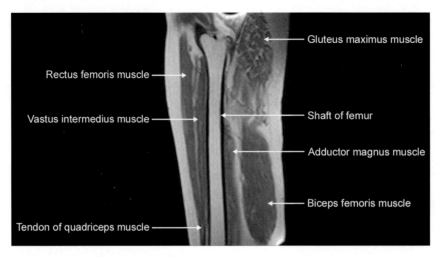

Fig. 9.11 Thigh MRI: Sagittal T1WI (corresponds to level 4 in Fig. 9.7)

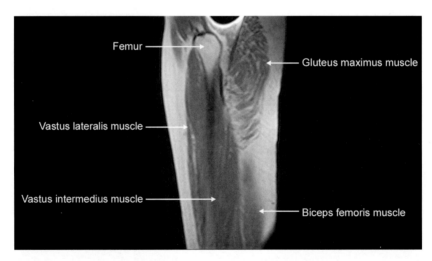

Fig. 9.12 Thigh MRI: Sagittal T1WI (corresponds to level 5 in Fig. 9.7)

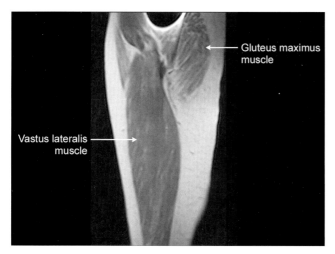

Fig. 9.13 Thigh MRI: Sagittal T1WI (corresponds to level 6 in Fig. 9.7)

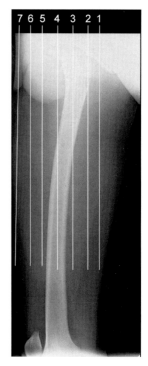

Fig. 9.14 Thigh MRI: Coronal section plan

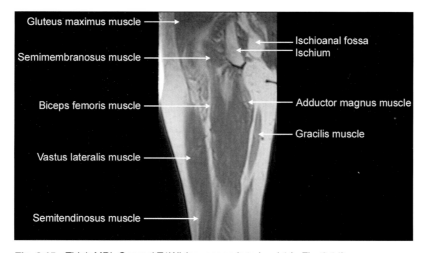

Fig. 9.15 Thigh MRI: Coronal T1WI (corresponds to level 1 in Fig. 9.14)

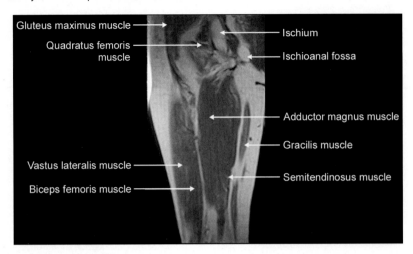

Fig. 9.16 Thigh MRI: Coronal T1WI (corresponds to level 2 in Fig. 9.14)

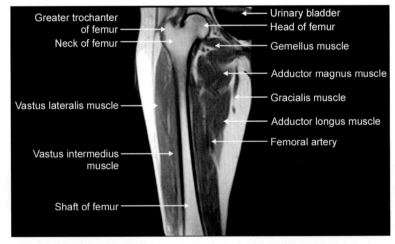

Fig. 9.17 Thigh MRI: Coronal T1WI (corresponds to level 3 in Fig. 9.14)

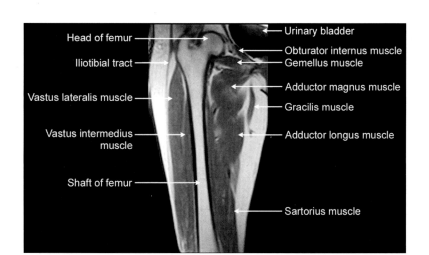

Fig. 9.18 Thigh MRI: Coronal T1WI (corresponds to level 4 in Fig. 9.14)

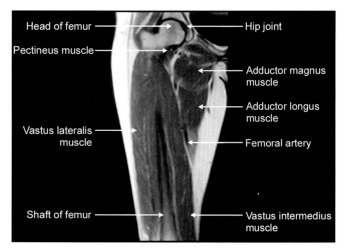

Fig. 9.19 Thigh MRI: Coronal T1WI (corresponds to level 5 in Fig. 9.14)

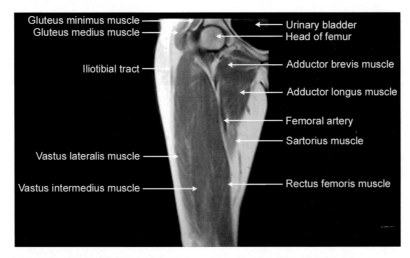

Fig. 9.20 Thigh MRI: Coronal T1WI (corresponds to level 6 in Fig. 9.14)

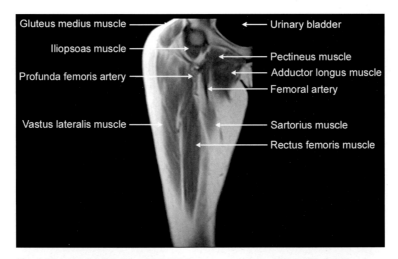

Fig. 9.21 Thigh MRI: Coronal T1WI (corresponds to level 7 in Fig. 9.14)

CHAPTER 10

Knee Joint

The knee joint is a modified pivotal hinge joint. It is the largest synovial joint in the body. It consists of two condylar joints between the femur and the tibia and a saddle joint between the patella and the femur. The intercondylar eminence of the tibia prevents sideway slipping of femur on tibia. The ligaments and muscles make knee a very stable joint.

The medial and lateral articular surfaces of the femur and tibia are asymmetrical. The distal surface of the medial condyle of the femur is narrower and more curved than the lateral condyle. The articular surface of lateral tibia is almost circular whereas the medial surface is oval in shape. The

articular surface of patella has a larger lateral and a smaller medial surface.

Inferiorly, the capsule is attached to the margins of the tibial condyles posteriorly except where the popliteus tendon cross the bone. On either sides the capsule is attached to the margins of the tibial condyles, and laterally to the head of the fibula. On its deeper aspect the coronary ligaments connect the capsule to the rims of menisci. The capsule is attached to the tibial tuberosity anteriorly on the tibia.

The ligaments of knee joint include the cruciate ligaments, arcuate popliteal ligament, the oblique popliteal ligament, fibular collateral ligament and the tibial collateral ligament.

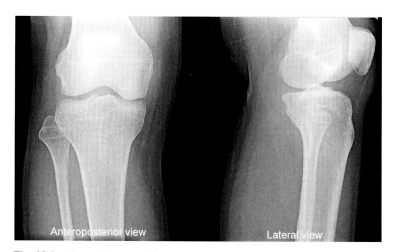

Anteroposterior view

Lateral view

Fig. 10.1 Knee joint

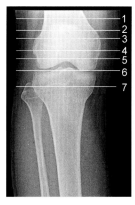

Fig. 10.2 Knee joint: Axial
section plan

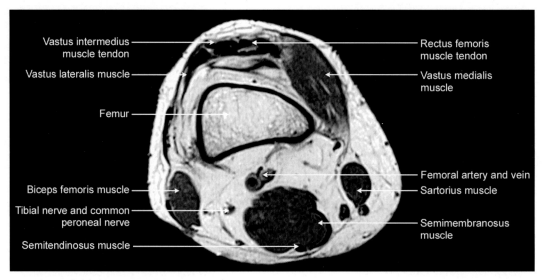

Fig. 10.3 Knee joint MRI: Axial T1WI (corresponds to level 1 in Fig. 10.2)

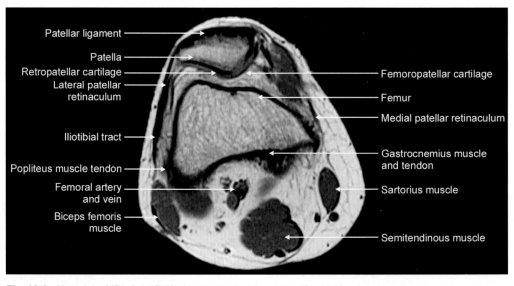

Fig. 10.4 Knee joint MRI: Axial T1WI (corresponds to level 2 in Fig. 10.2)

The cruciate ligaments are a pair of ligaments (anterior and posterior), they cross each other connecting the tibia to the femur and lie within the capsule of knee joint but outside the synovial membrane. The anterior cruciate ligament is attached to the anterior part of the tibial plateau between the attachments of anterior horns of medial and lateral menisci. Posteriorly, the anterior cruciate ligament is attached to the posteromedial aspect of lateral femoral condyle. The anterior cruciate ligament appears as a fan shaped structure, it is 11 mm wide and 31-38 mm long. The posterior cruciate ligament is attached posteriorly to the intercondylar area on tibia and anteriorly it is attached to the anterolateral aspect of the medial femoral condyle. The posterior cruciate ligament is about 13 mm wide and about 38 mm long. Both these ligaments stabilize the knee in a rotational fashion. Thus, if one of these ligaments is significantly damaged, the knee will be unstable when planting the foot of the injured extremity and pivoting, causes the knee to buckle and give way.

The arcuate popliteal ligament is a Y-shaped thickening of posterior capsular fibers, the stem of the Y is attached to the head of fibula. The medial limb of Y is attached to the posterior edge of the intercondylar area, while the lateral limb is attached to the lateral femoral condyle.

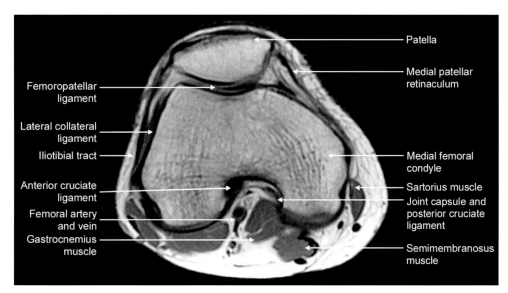

Fig. 10.5   Knee joint MRI: Axial T1WI (corresponds to level 3 in Fig. 10.2)

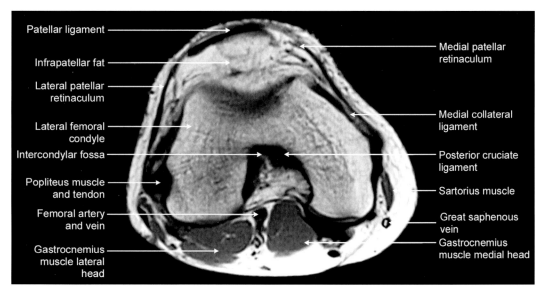

Fig. 10.6   Knee joint MRI: Axial T1WI (corresponds to level 4 in Fig. 10.2)

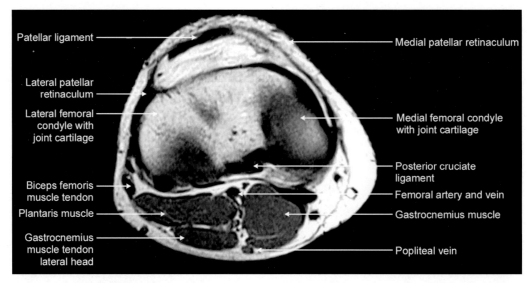

Fig. 10.7 Knee joint MRI: Axial T1WI (corresponds to level 5 in Fig. 10.2)

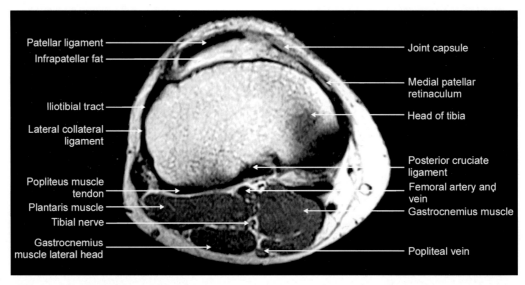

Fig. 10.8 Knee joint MRI: Axial T1WI (corresponds to level 6 in Fig. 10.2)

The oblique popliteal ligament is an expansion of the tendon of semimembranosus muscle that blends with the capsule posteriorly and ascends laterally.

The tibial collateral ligament is a triangular band 8-9 cm in length, attached above to the medial femoral epicondyle and below to the medial surface of tibia. Its anterior margin forms the vertical base of the triangle and is free except at its attached

extremities. The posterior apex of the triangular ligament blends with the capsule and is also attached to the medial meniscus.

The fibular collateral ligament is 'cord-like' and is attached superiorly to the lateral epicondyle and inferiorly to the head of the fibula.

The patellar ligament is a central band of the tendon of quadriceps femoris muscles; it is about 8 cm long. Proximally, it

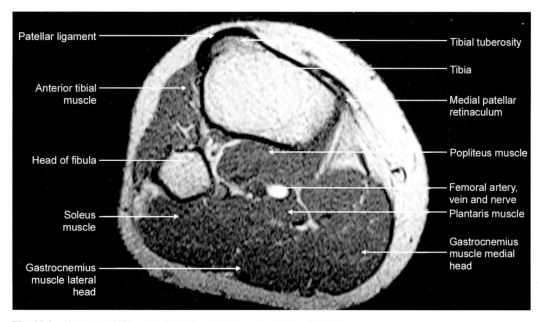

Patellar ligament

Anterior tibial
muscle

Head of fibula

Soleus
muscle

Gastrocnemius
muscle lateral
head

Tibial tuberosity

Tibia

Medial patellar
retinaculum

Popliteus muscle

Femoral artery,
vein and nerve

Plantaris muscle

Gastrocnemius
muscle medial
head

Fig. 10.9 Knee joint MRI: Axial T1WI (corresponds to level 7 in Fig. 10.2)

attaches to the anterior and posterior surfaces of patella including the apex. Distally it attaches to the smooth area of tibial tuberosity. The patellar ligament blends with the medial and lateral patellar retinaculum, which are aponeurotic expansions of vastus medialis and lateralis. The retinaculum supports the articular capsule of the knee laterally.

The menisci are called semilunar cartilages. These are cresenteric disks of fibrocartilage that act as shock absorbers. The menisci are avascular structures comprising mainly of collagenous fibrous tissue attached to the tibial plateau. There are two menisci, the lateral and the medial meniscus. They are triangular in cross-section, being thicker at their convex periphery (5 mm in height). Their distal surfaces are flat while their proximal surfaces are concave and articulate with the convex femoral condyles. The menisci demonstrate diffusely low signal on all MRI pulse sequences because of their fibrocartilaginous nature.

The medial menisci is almost a semicircle in appearance and is broader posteriorly. Its anterior horn is attached to the intercondylar area in front of the anterior cruciate ligament; the posterior horn is attached in front of the posterior cruciate ligament in intercondylar area. The lateral meniscus is of uniform width and almost forms a complete circle. Its anterior horn is attached in front of the intercondylar eminence of the tibia behind the anterior cruciate ligament, while the

posterior horn is attached in front of the posterior horn of the medial meniscus.

The synovial membrane lines the internal surface of the fibrous capsule and attaches to the periphery of the patella and the edges of the menisci. The synovial membrane is continuous with the lining of the suprapatellar bursa. Normal amount of synovial fluid is 0.5 ml.

Bursae of knee joint reduce the friction between tendon and bones. The suprapatellar bursa lies between the femur and the quadriceps femoris. The prepatellar bursa lies between the skin and the patella. The infrapatellar bursa lies between the skin and the tibial tuberosity. The deep infrapatellar bursa lies between the patellar ligament and the upper part of the tibia. The semimembranosus bursa lies between that muscle and the medial head of gastrocnemius.

Blood supply to knee joint is by anastomosis of the genicular branches of the popliteal artery. The middle genicular branches supply the cruciate ligaments.

Movements at the knee joint are the flexion, extension and rotation. Flexion is limited to about 150 degrees due to soft parts behind the knee. Flexion movements are primarily performed by the hamstring muscles. Extension is performed by the quadriceps femoris muscles assisted by tensor fascia lata. As the knee extends the shorter and rounded lateral femoral condyle completes its extension to about 30 degrees short of

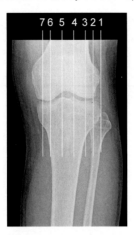

Fig. 10.10   Knee joint MRI: Sagittal section plan

full extension. The rotation movement occurs during extension with the foot on ground. Passive medial rotation of the femur is a part of a 'locking' mechanism which secures the joint in 5-10 degrees of hyperextension when both the cruciate ligaments, the collateral ligaments and the oblique popliteal ligament are all taut. Lateral rotation is produced by the popliteus muscle when flexion occurs with the foot free.

The knee joint is stabilized by the surrounding muscles and their tendons. Anteriorly, it is the quadriceps tendon. This broad tendon attaches to and surrounds the patella and continues as the patellar ligament, which is attached to the tuberosity of the tibia. Posteriorly are the popliteus, plantaris and medial and lateral heads of gastrocnemius. Laterally are the tendons of the biceps femoris and popliteus. Medially by the sartorius, gracilis, semitendinosus and semimembranosus muscles.

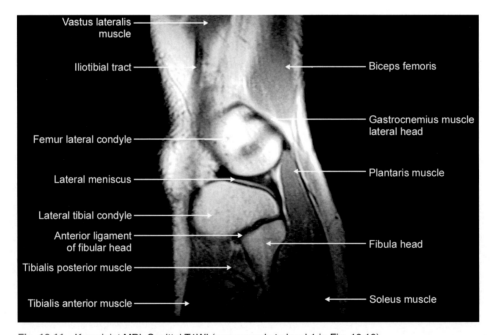

Fig. 10.11   Knee joint MRI: Sagittal T1WI (corresponds to level 1 in Fig. 10.10)

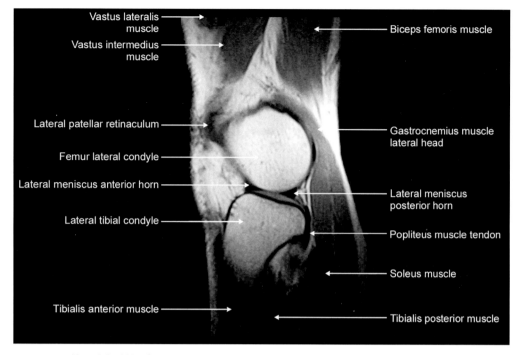

Fig. 10.12 Knee joint MRI: Sagittal T1WI (corresponds to level 2 in Fig. 10.10)

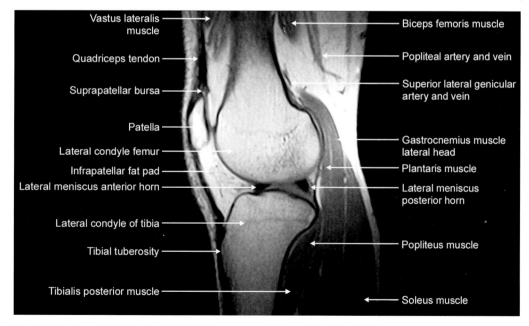

Fig. 10.13 Knee joint MRI: Sagittal T1WI (corresponds to level 3 in Fig. 10.10)

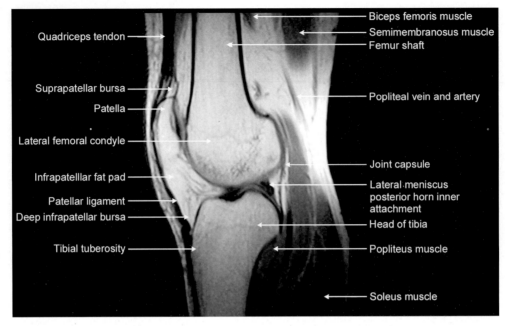

Quadriceps tendon

Suprapatellar bursa

Patella

Lateral femoral condyle

Infrapatelllar fat pad

Patellar ligament

Deep infrapatellar bursa

Tibial tuberosity

Biceps femoris muscle

Semimembranosus muscle

Femur shaft

Popliteal vein and artery

Joint capsule

Lateral meniscus posterior horn inner attachment

Head of tibia

Popliteus muscle

Soleus muscle

Fig. 10.14   Knee joint MRI: Sagittal T1WI (corresponds to level 4 in Fig. 10.10)

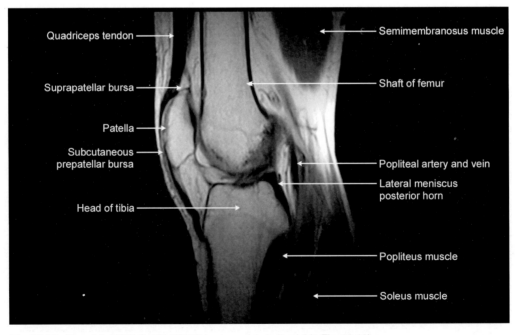

Quadriceps tendon

Suprapatellar bursa

Patella

Subcutaneous prepatellar bursa

Head of tibia

Semimembranosus muscle

Shaft of femur

Popliteal artery and vein

Lateral meniscus posterior horn

Popliteus muscle

Soleus muscle

Fig. 10.15   Knee joint MRI: Sagittal T1WI (corresponds to level 5 in Fig. 10.10)

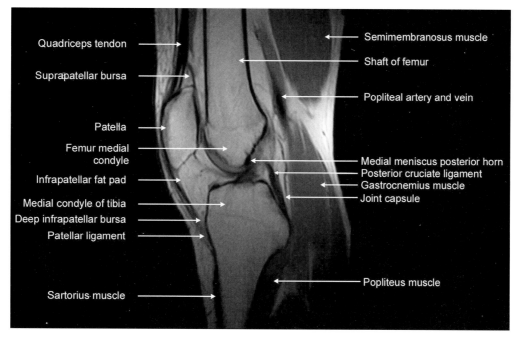

Quadriceps tendon

Suprapatellar bursa

Patella

Femur medial condyle

Infrapatellar fat pad

Medial condyle of tibia

Deep infrapatellar bursa

Patellar ligament

Sartorius muscle

Semimembranosus muscle

Shaft of femur

Popliteal artery and vein

Medial meniscus posterior horn
Posterior cruciate ligament
Gastrocnemius muscle
Joint capsule

Popliteus muscle

Fig. 10.16   Knee joint MRI: Sagittal T1WI (corresponds to level 6 in Fig. 10.10)

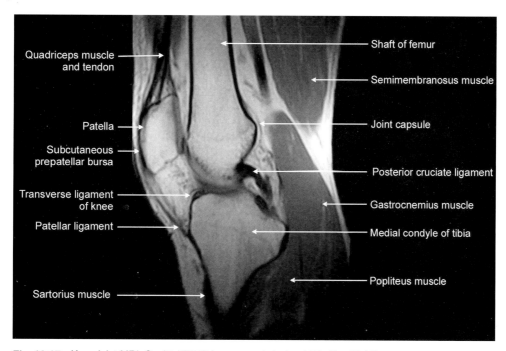

Quadriceps muscle and tendon

Patella

Subcutaneous prepatellar bursa

Transverse ligament of knee

Patellar ligament

Sartorius muscle

Shaft of femur

Semimembranosus muscle

Joint capsule

Posterior cruciate ligament

Gastrocnemius muscle

Medial condyle of tibia

Popliteus muscle

Fig. 10.17   Knee joint MRI: Sagittal T1WI (corresponds to level 7 in Fig. 10.10)

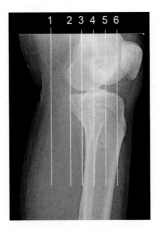

Fig. 10.18   Knee joint coronal section plan

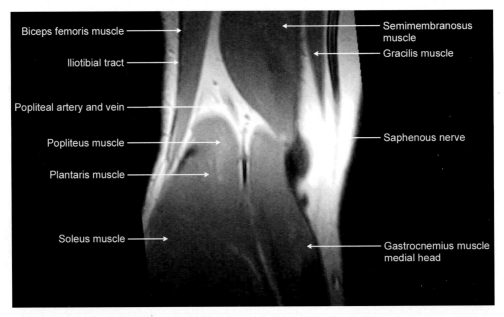

Fig. 10.19   Knee joint MRI: Coronal T1WI (corresponds to level 1 in Fig. 10.18)

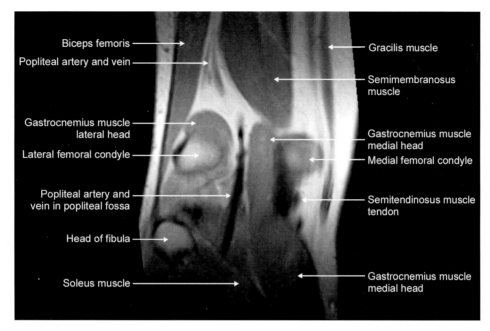

Biceps femoris
Popliteal artery and vein
Gastrocnemius muscle lateral head
Lateral femoral condyle
Popliteal artery and vein in popliteal fossa
Head of fibula
Soleus muscle

Gracilis muscle
Semimembranosus muscle
Gastrocnemius muscle medial head
Medial femoral condyle
Semitendinosus muscle tendon
Gastrocnemius muscle medial head

Fig. 10.20   Knee joint MRI: Coronal T1WI (corresponds to level 2 in Fig. 10.18)

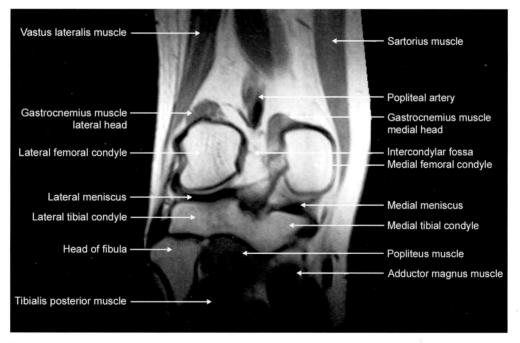

Vastus lateralis muscle
Gastrocnemius muscle lateral head
Lateral femoral condyle
Lateral meniscus
Lateral tibial condyle
Head of fibula
Tibialis posterior muscle

Sartorius muscle
Popliteal artery
Gastrocnemius muscle medial head
Intercondylar fossa
Medial femoral condyle
Medial meniscus
Medial tibial condyle
Popliteus muscle
Adductor magnus muscle

Fig. 10.21   Knee joint MRI: Coronal T1WI (corresponds to level 3 in Fig. 10.18)

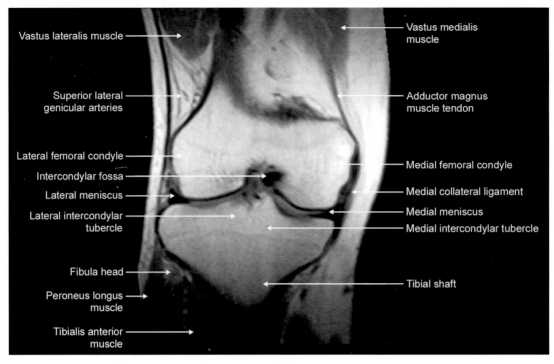

Fig. 10.22   Knee joint MRI: Coronal T1WI (corresponds to level 4 in Fig. 10.18)

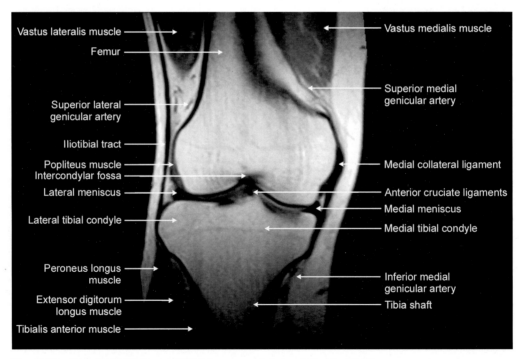

Fig. 10.23   Knee joint MRI: Coronal T1WI (corresponds to level 5 in Fig. 10.18)

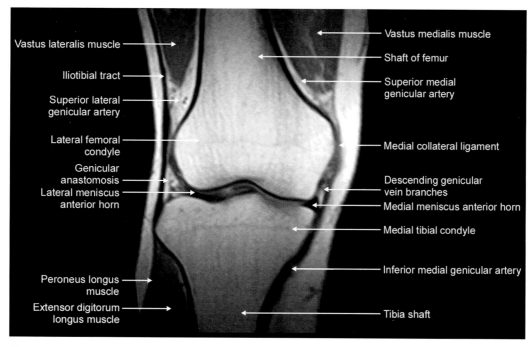

Fig. 10.24 Knee joint MRI: Coronal T1WI (corresponds to level 6 in Fig. 10.18)

CHAPTER 11

Leg

Muscles of the anterior compartment of leg are: tibialis anterior, extensor hallucis longus, extensor digitorum longus and peroneus tertius muscle. The tibialis anterior muscle is attached to the lateral condyle and superior half of lateral surface of tibia, distally the muscle is attached to the medial cuneiform and base of first metatarsal. It is innervated by the deep fibular nerve. The main action of tibialis anterior muscle is dorsiflexion at ankle and inversion of foot.

The extensor hallucis longus and extensor digitorum longus originate from the anterior surfaces of tibia and fibula and the anterior surface of the interosseous membrane. The extensor hallucis longus inserts into the dorsal aspect of base of distal phalanx of great toe. The extensor digitorum longus inserts into the middle and distal phalanges of lateral four digits. The main action of these muscles is to extend the great toe and the four lateral digits. The peroneus tertius muscle originates from the inferior surface of anterior

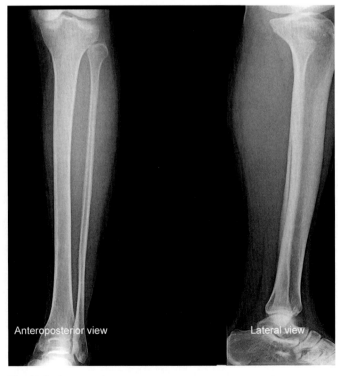

Fig. 11.1 Leg

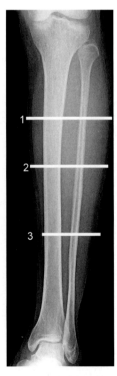

Fig. 11.2 Leg MRI: Axial section plan

surface of fibula and interosseous membrane and inserts into the dorsum of base of fifth metatarsal. Its main action is to dorsiflex the ankle and eversion of foot. These muscles are innervated by the L5 and S1 nerves.

Muscles of the lateral compartment of leg are: peroneus longus muscle, peroneus brevis muscles. These muscles originate from the superior, inferior and lateral surfaces of the head of fibula. The peroneus longus muscle inserts into the base of first metatarsal and medial cuneiform. The peroneus brevis inserts into the dorsal surface of fifth metatarsal. Both these muscles are innervated by the superficial peroneal nerve (L5, S1 and S2). Their main action is eversion of the foot and plantar flexion of the ankle.

Posterior compartment of leg has two broad groups – the superficial group and deep group of muscles. The superficial group comprises of gastrocnemius, soleus and plantaris. The

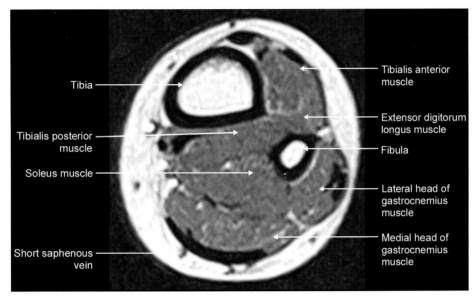

Fig. 11.3   Leg MRI: Axial T1WI (corresponds to level 1 in Fig. 11.2)

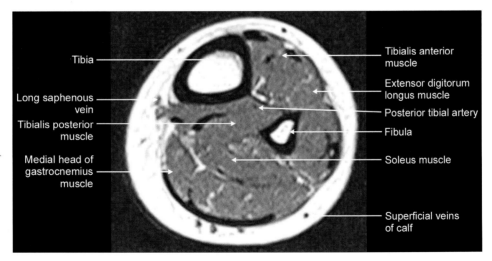

Fig. 11.4   Leg MRI: Axial T1WI (corresponds to level 2 in Fig. 11.2)

gastrocnemius muscle has two heads—the lateral head originates from the lateral condyle of femur and the medial head arises from medial condyle of femur. The soleus arises from the posterior aspect of head of fibula, posterior surface of fibula and medial border of tibia. Both gastroneminus and soleus muscles inserted into the posterior surface of calcaneus as the tendocalcaneus. They are innervated by the tibial nerve (S1 and S2). Their main action is to plantar flexion of the ankle and flexion of leg at knee joint. The plantaris muscle originates from inferior end of lateral supracondylar line of femur and oblique popliteal ligament. Its main action is to assist in plantar flexion of ankle and flexion at knee joint.

The deep group of muscles are popliteus, flexor hallucis longus, flexor digitorum longus, tibialis posterior muscles. The popliteus muscle originates from the lateral surface of lateral condyle of femur and lateral meniscus and inserts into the posterior surface of tibia. It is innervated by the tibial nerve (L4, L5 and S1), its main action is flexion at knee joint. Flexor hallucis longus originates from posterior surface of fibula and inferior part of interosseous membrane to insert distally into the base of distal phalanx of great toe. Its main action is flexion at great toe and plantar flexion at ankle. It also supports the medial longitudinal arch of foot. The flexor digitorum longus originates from medial part of posterior surface of tibia and fibula to insert distally into the bases of distal phalanges of lateral four digits. Its main action is flexion of lateral four digits and plantar flexion of ankle. Both the flexor digitorum longus muscle and flexor hallucis longus muscle are innervated by tibial nerve (S2 and S3). The tibialis posterior muscle origi-

nates from the interosseous membrane and the posterior surfaces of tibia and fibula, it is attached distally to the tuberosity of navicular, cuneiform, cuboid and bases of second, third and fourth metatarsals. Its main action is plantar flexion of ankle and inversion of the foot. It is innervated by the tibial nerve (L4 and L5).

Arterial supply of leg is by the popliteal artery, anterior and posterior tibial arteries and peroneal artery. The popliteal artery is the continuation of femoral artery in adductor canal. The popliteal artery courses in the popliteal fossa deep to the popliteal vein and divides into the anterior and posterior tibial arteries at the lower border of popliteus muscle. The popliteal artery gives off the superior, middle and inferior genicular branches to the lateral and medial aspects of knee. The anterior tibial artery passes between the tibia and fibula into the anterior compartment through an opening in the superior part of interosseous membrane and continues downwards between tibialis anterior and extensor digitorum longus muscles and supplies the anterior compartment of leg. The peroneal artery originates from posterior tibial artery; it descends in the posterior compartment adjacent to posterior intermuscular septum. The peroneal artery supplies the posterior compartment of leg and its perforating branches supply the lateral aspect of leg. The posterior tibial artery passes through the posterior compartment of the leg and terminates distal to the flexor retinaculum by dividing into medial and lateral plantar arteries. The posterior tibial artery supplies the posterior and lateral compartments of leg, it also gives off the nutrient artery to tibia.

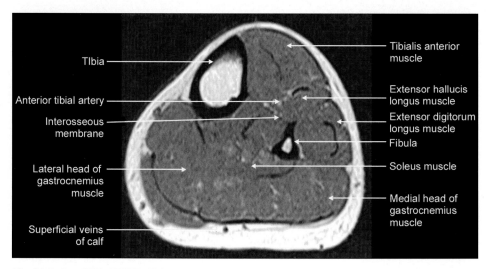

Fig. 11.5 Leg MRI: Axial T1WI (corresponds to level 3 in Fig. 11.2)

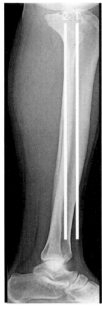

Fig. 11.6   Leg coronal section plan

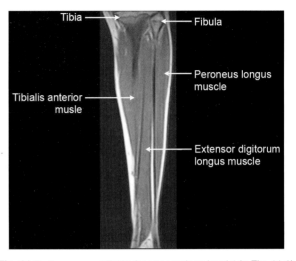

Fig. 11.7   Leg coronal T1WI (corresponds to level 1 in Fig. 11.6)

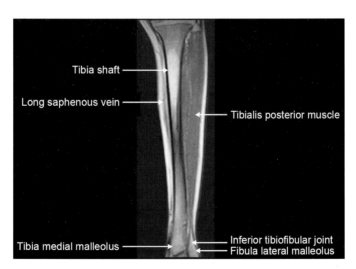

Fig. 11.8   Leg coronal T1WI (corresponds to level 2 in Fig. 11.6)

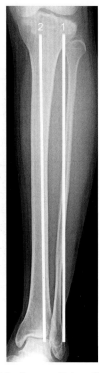

Fig. 11.9 Leg sagittal section plan

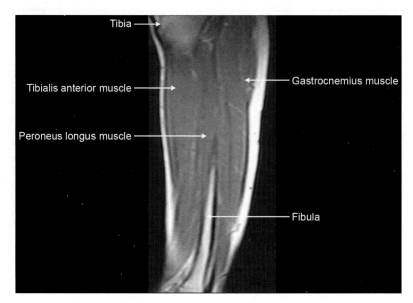

Fig. 11.10 Leg MRI: Sagittal T1WI (corresponds to level 1 in Fig. 11.9)

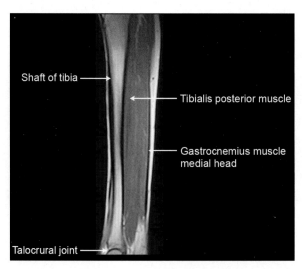

Fig. 11.11 Leg MRI: Sagittal T1WI (corresponds to level 2 in Fig. 11.9)

Ankle Joint

The ankle joint or the talocrural joint is constructed on four bones: the tibia, fibula, talus and calcaneum. The body weight is transmitted through the tibia to the talus which distributes anteriorly and posteriorly within the foot.

The ankle joint has two groups of ligaments—the lateral collateral ligaments and the medial collateral ligaments. These ligaments are strong fibrous bands and they are extremely important in the stability of the ankle joint.

The lateral collateral ligament prevents excessive inversion and comprises of anterior talofibular ligament, calcaneofibular ligament and posterior talofibular ligament.

The medial collateral ligament or the deltoid ligament is thicker than the lateral ligament and spreads in a fan shape manner to cover the distal end of the tibia and the inner surfaces of the talus, navicular, and calcaneus. The medial collateral ligament or deltoid ligament include the tibionavicular ligament, calcaneotibial ligament, anterior talotibial ligament and the posterior talotibial ligament. They prevent abduction and limit plantar flexion and dorsiflexion of the ankle joint.

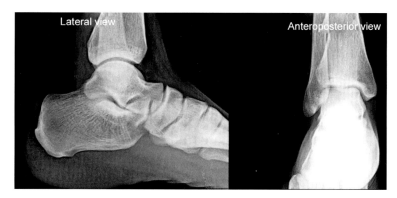

Fig. 12.1 Ankle joint

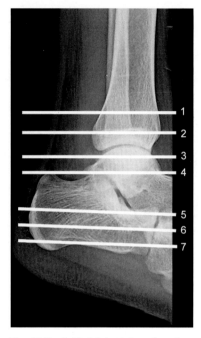

Fig. 12.2 Ankle joint axial section plan

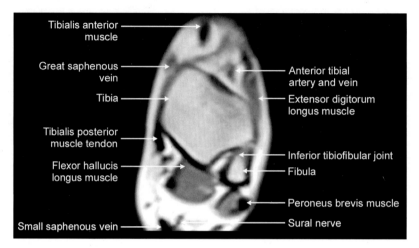

Fig. 12.3 Ankle joint MRI: Axial T1WI (corresponds to level 1 in Fig. 12.2)

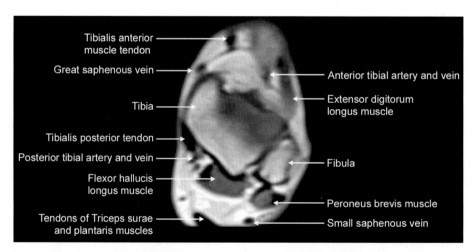

Fig. 12.4 Ankle joint MRI: Axial T1WI (corresponds to level 2 in Fig. 12.2)

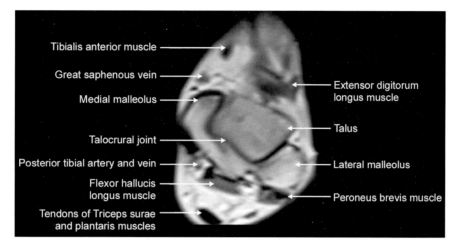

Fig. 12.5 Ankle joint MRI: Axial T1WI (corresponds to level 3 in Fig. 12.2)

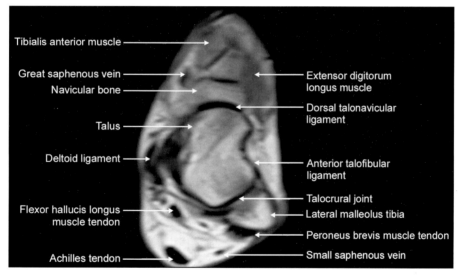

Fig. 12.6 Ankle joint MRI: Axial T1WI (corresponds to level 4 in Fig. 12.2)

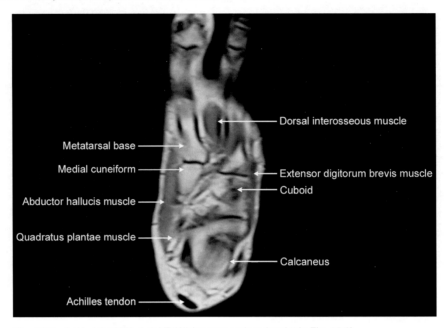

Fig. 12.7   Ankle joint MRI: Axial T1WI (corresponds to level 5 in Fig. 12.2)

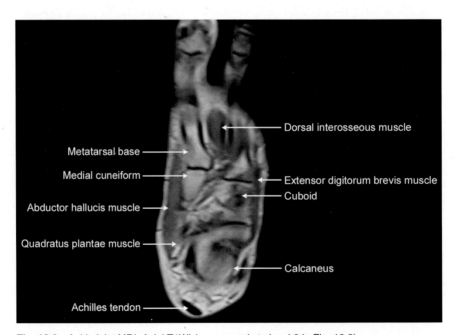

Fig. 12.8   Ankle joint MRI: Axial T1WI (corresponds to level 6 in Fig. 12.2)

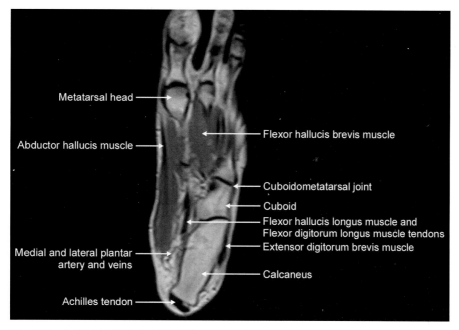

Fig. 12.9 Ankle joint MRI: Axial T1WI (corresponds to level 7 in Fig. 12.2)

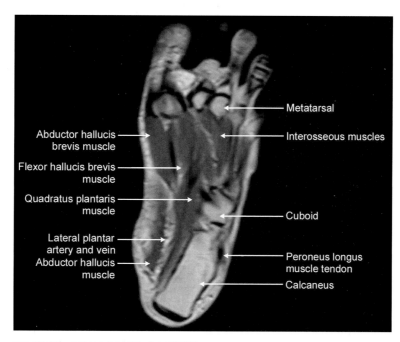

Fig. 12.10 Ankle joint MRI: Axial T1WI

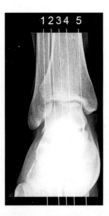

Fig. 12.11 Ankle joint sagittal section plan

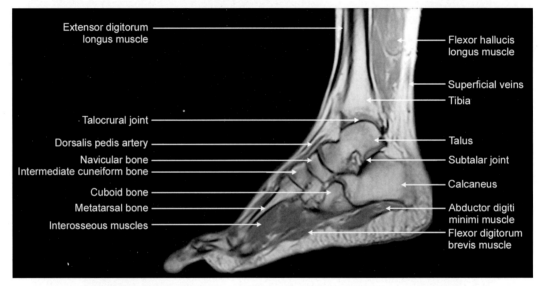

Fig. 12.12 Ankle joint MRI: Sagittal T1WI (corresponds to level 1 in Fig. 12.11)

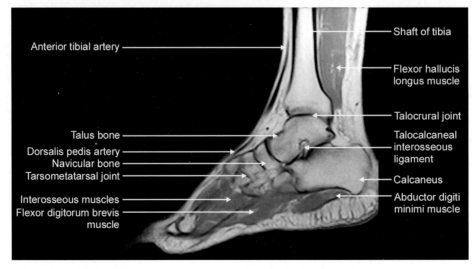

Fig. 12.13 Ankle joint MRI: Sagittal T1WI (corresponds to level 2 in Fig. 12.11)

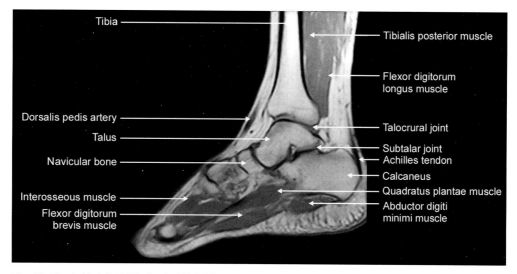

Fig. 12.14 Ankle joint MRI: Sagittal T1WI (corresponds to level 3 in Fig. 12.11)

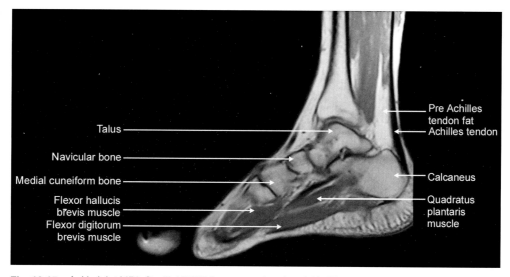

Fig. 12.15 Ankle joint MRI: Sagittal T1WI (corresponds to level 4 in Fig. 12.11)

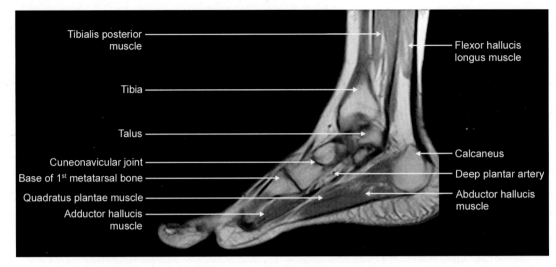

Fig. 12.16 Ankle joint MRI: Sagittal T1WI (corresponds to level 5 in Fig. 12.11)

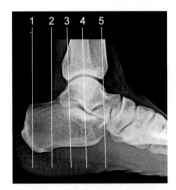

Fig. 12.17 Ankle joint coronal section plan

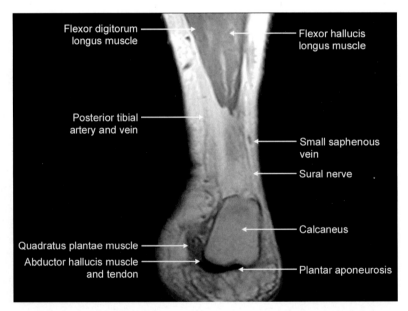

Fig. 12.18 Ankle joint MRI: Coronal T1WI (corresponds to level 1 in Fig. 12.17)

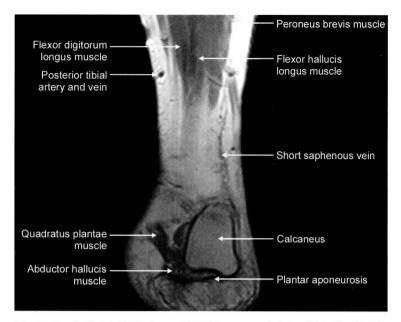

Fig. 12.19 Ankle joint MRI: Coronal T1WI (corresponds to level 2 in Fig. 12.17)

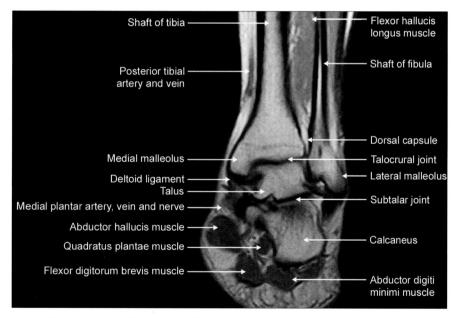

Fig. 12.20 Ankle joint MRI: Coronal T1WI (corresponds to level 3 in Fig. 12.17)

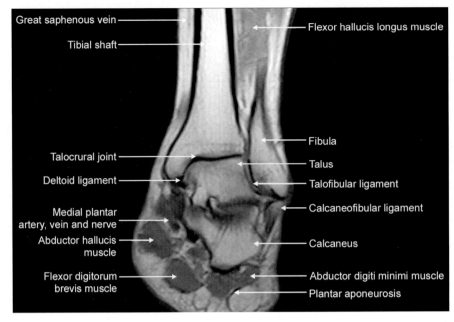

Fig. 12.21 Ankle joint MRI: Coronal T1WI (corresponds to level 4 in Fig. 12.17)

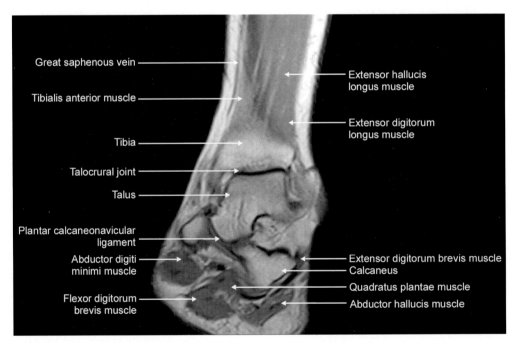

Fig. 12.22 Ankle joint MRI: Coronal T1WI (corresponds to level 5 in Fig. 12.17)

CHAPTER 13

MRI Contrast

Intravenous Contrast Agents

In MRI, the most commonly used intravenous contrast agents are gadolinium chelates, the paramagnetic property of gadolinium provides contrast. It has the ability to alter the magnetic characteristics of neighboring tissues. The effect of this is shortening of the T1 and T2 relaxation times. Shortening of T1 effects are exploited since shortening of T1 relaxation time leads to an increase in signal intensity.

Gadolinium containing contrast agents available are gadodiamide (Omniscan), gadobenic acid (Multihance), gadopentetic acid (Magnevist), gadoteridol (Prohance), gadofosveset (Ablavar), gadoversetamide (OptiMARK), gadoxetic acid (Eovist or Primovist).

Other MRI contrast agents gaining recognition are superparamagnetic agents, i.e. iron oxide and manganese.

Two types of iron oxide contrast agents exist: Superparamagnetic Iron Oxide (SPIO) and Ultrasmall Superparamagnetic Iron Oxide (USPIO). These contrast agents consist of suspended colloids of iron oxide nanoparticles and are injectables, they reduce the T2 signals of absorbing tissues. SPIO and USPIO contrast agents have been used successfully in some liver tumor enhancement. Available iron oxide contrast agents are Cliavist, Combidex, Resovist and Sinerem.

Manganese chelates such as Mn-DPDP enhance the T1 signal and have been used for the detection of liver lesions. It is absorbed intracellularly and excreted in bile.

Oral Contrast Agents

In MRI oral contrast can be used for enhancement of the gastrointestinal tract. Gadolinium, manganese chelates and iron salts are used for T1 signal enhancement.

SPIO, barium sulfate, air and clay have been used to lower T2 signal. Blueberry and green tea having high manganese concentration can also be used for T1 increasing contrast enhancement.

Perflubron, a type of perfluorocarbon, has been used as a gastrointestinal MRI contrast agent for pediatric imaging. This contrast agent works by reducing the amount of protons in a body cavity.

Gadolinium initially disperses through the vascular system and then diffuses into the extracellular space, before moving into the intracellular space. Whilst still circulating within the vessels, magnetic resonance angiography (MRA) can be performed.

Gadolinium does not cross the intact blood-brain barrier but helps identifying intracranial lesions with interruption of the barrier, like infection and tumors. It helps to discriminate tumors from edema, low-grade from high-grade tumors, scar tissue from a tumor tissue.

Oral gadolinium is used to highlight loops of bowel to distinguish from surrounding soft tissue.

Superparamagnetic agents are more specific hepatic agent and are specially taken up by the Kupffer cells in the liver and help make a distinction between normal liver and malignant tissue.

MRA

All pulse sequences are sensitive to flow. There is a complex relationship between the type and rate of flow and the resultant signal intensity. As a general rule, fast or turbulent vascular flow results in a signal dropout, whilst slow vascular flow results in high signal. There are two principal flow-sensitive sequences, time of flight and phase contrast. MRA can also be performed with intravenous gadolinium whilst in the vascular phase of enhancement.

CHAPTER **14**

Ossification Centers

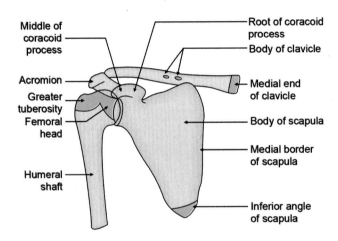

Fig. 14.1 Shoulder joint

Labels in figure:
- Middle of coracoid process
- Acromion
- Greater tuberosity
- Femoral head
- Humeral shaft
- Root of coracoid process
- Body of clavicle
- Medial end of clavicle
- Body of scapula
- Medial border of scapula
- Inferior angle of scapula

Table 14.1	Shoulder joint	
Bones	**Ossification**	
Body of scapula	8th Week of fetal life	
Body of clavicle (two centers)	5th and 6th Week of fetal life	
Shaft of humerus	8th Week of fetal life	
Epiphysis	**Appearance**	**Fusion**
Head of humerus	1 year	
Greater tuberosity	3 years	
Lesser tuberosity	5 years	
Acromion process	15–18 years	25th year
Middle of coracoid process	1 year	15th year
Root of coracoid process	17th years	25th year
Inferior angle of scapula	14–20 years	22–25 years
Medial border of scapula	14–20 years	22–25 years
Medial end of clavicle	18–20 years	25th year

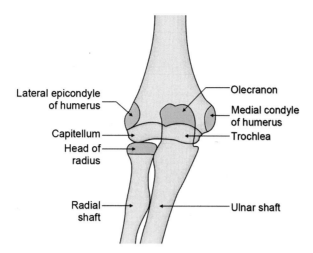

Fig. 14.2   Elbow joint

Table 14.2	Elbow joint	
Bones	**Ossification**	
Radial shaft	8th Week of fetal life	
Ulnar shaft	8th Week of fetal life	
Epiphysis	**Appearance**	**Fusion**
Lateral epicondyle	10–12 years	17–18 years
Medial epicondyle	05–08 years	17–18 years
Capitellum	01–03 years	17–18 years
Head of radius	05–06 years	16–19 years
Trochlea	11th year	18th year
Olecranon process	10–13 years	16–20 years

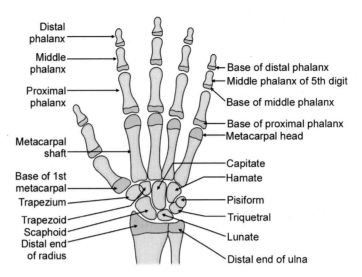

Fig. 14.3   Wrist and hand

Table 14.3	Wrist and hand

Bones	Ossification	
Capitate	4 months	
Hamate	4 months	
Triquetral	3 years	
Lunate	4–5 years	
Trapezium	6 years	
Trapezoid	6 years	
Capitate	6 years	
Scaphoid	6 years	
Pisiform	11 years	
Metacarpals	10th Week of fetal life	
Proximal phalanges	11th Week of fetal life	
Middle phalanges	12th Week of fetal life	
Distal phalanges	9th Week of fetal life	
Middle phalanx of 5th digit	14th Week of fetal life	
Epiphysis	**Appearance**	**Fusion**
Lower end of radius	1–2 years	20th year
Lower end of ulna	5–8 years	20th year
Metacarpal heads	2.5 years	20th year
Base of proximal phalanges	2.5 years	20th year
Base of middle phalanges	3 years	18–20 years
Base of distal phalanges	3 years	18–20 years
Base of 1st metacarpal	2.5 years	20th year

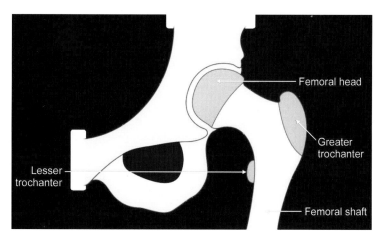

Fig. 14.4   Hip joint

Table 14.4	Hip joint	
Bones	**Ossification**	
Proximal femoral shaft	7th Week of fetal life	
Epiphysis	**Appearance**	**Fusion**
Femoral head	1 year	18–20 years
Greater trochanter	3–5 years	18–20 years
Lesser trochanter	8–14 years	18–20 years

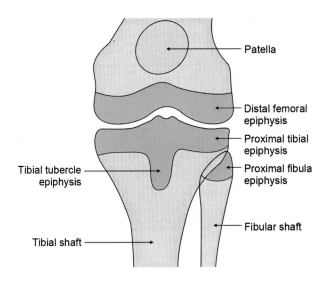

Fig. 14.5 Knee joint

Table 14.5	Knee joint	
Bones	**Ossification**	
Tibial shaft	7th Week of fetal life	
Fibular shaft	8th Week of fetal life	
Patella	5 years	
Epiphysis	**Appearance**	**Fusion**
Proximal tibia	At birth	20th year
Tibial tubercle	5–10 years	20th year
Proximal fibular	4th year	25th year
Distal femur	At birth	20th year

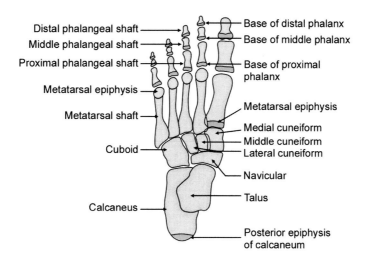

Fig. 14.6   Foot

| Table 14.6 | Foot |

Bones	Ossification
Calcaneus	6th Month of fetal life
Talus	6th Month of fetal life
Navicular	3–4 years
Cuboid	At birth
Lateral cuneiform	1 year
Middle cuneiform	3 years
Medial cuneiform	3 years
Metatarsal shafts	8th–9th Week of fetal life
Phalangeal shafts	10th Week of fetal life

Epiphysis	Appearance	Fusion
Metatarsals	3 years	17–20 years
Proximal phalangeal base	3 years	17–20 years
Middle phalangeal base	3 years	17–20 years
Distal phalangeal base	5 years	17–20 years
Posterior calcaneal	5 years	At puberty

CHAPTER **15**

Magnetic Resonance-Positron Emission Tomography (MR-PET)

P rototypes of integrated MR systems (Fig. 15.1) that can produce simultaneous, integrated images of the brain (Fig. 15.2) are currently under development and not commercially available. MRI gives structural details and provides high soft tissue resolution images whereas positron emission tomography (PET) uses a radioactive tracer in the body to obtain functional information of a particular organ or system, locate metastasis, recurrence of tumors and help in determining the effectiveness of treatment in malignant diseases. However, PET gives molecular detail but fails to give anatomical information. The combined capability of MR-PET has been developed. While PET evaluates the metabolic aspects, MRI gives high resolution anatomical information.

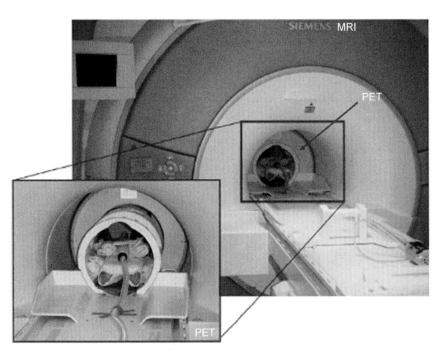

Fig. 15.1 MR-PET equipment, in this each scan occurs without repositioning the patient (*Courtesy:* Siemens Ag., Germany) *(For color version, see Plate 1)*

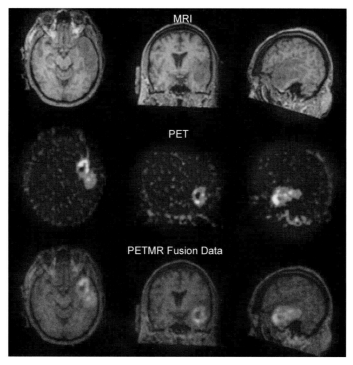

Fig. 15.2 MR-PET and fusion images demonstrates the glioma proliferation (*Courtesy:* Siemens Ag., Germany) *(For color version, see Plate 1)*

MR-PET gains over PET-CT are that MR-PET provides excellent soft tissue image and the patient is not exposed to radiations. PET-MRI can differentiate tumor recurrence from fibrosis following radiotherapy.

MR-PET is a modality with tremendous potential for combining structure and function. The images of MR-PET are useful to diagnose intricate cases, planning and treatment and follow-up. In addition to imaging tumors and conducting functional studies, MR-PET may lead to increased understanding of diseases like Alzheimer's, Parkinson's, stroke, depression, schizophrenia, and could even help in refining surgery. MR-PET once available will revolutionize the field of medicine on treatment and follow up of cases.

CHAPTER 16

Picture Archiving and Communication System

Picture archiving and communication system (PACS), is based on universal DICOM (Digital imaging and communications in medicine) format. DICOM solutions are capable of storing and retrieving multi modality images in a proficient and secure manner in assisting and improving hospital workflow and patient diagnosis.

The aim of PACS is to replace conventional radiographs and reports with a completely electronic network, these digital images can be viewed on monitors in the radiology department, emergency rooms, inpatient and outpatient departments, thus saving time, improving efficiency of hospital and avoid incurring the cost of hard copy images in a busy hospital. The three basic means of rendering plain radiographs images to digital are computed radiography (CR) using photostimulable phosphor plate technology; direct digital radiography (DDR) and digitizing conventional analog films. Nonimage data, such as scanned documents like PDF (portable document format) is also incorporated in DICOM format. Dictation of reports can

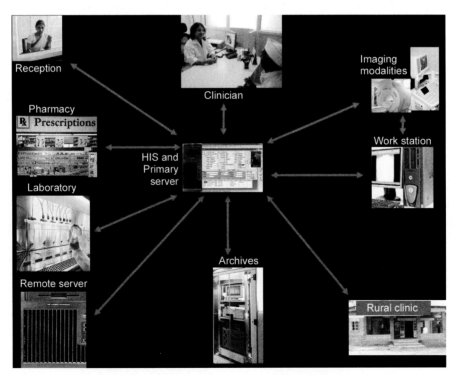

Fig. 16.1   Picture Archiving and Communication System (PACS) Flow chart
(For color version, see Plate 2)

be integrated into the system. The recording is automatically sent to a transcript writer's workstation for typing, but it can also be made available for access by physicians, avoiding typing delays for urgent results.

Radiology has led the way in developing PACS to its present high standards. PACS consists of four major components: the imaging modalities such as radiography, computed radiography, endoscopy, mammography, ultrasound, CT, PET-CT and MRI, a secured network for the transmission of patient information, workstations for interpreting and reviewing images and archives for the storage and retrieval of images and reports. Backup copies of patient images are made provisioned in case the image is lost from the PACS. There are several methods for backup storage of images, but they typically involve automatically sending copies of the images to a separate computer for storage, preferably off-site.

In PACS no patient is irradiated simply because a previous radiograph or CT scan has been lost; the image once acquired onto the PACS is always available when needed. Simultaneous multilocation viewing of the same image is possible on any workstation connected to the PACS. Numerous post processing soft copy manipulations are possible on the viewing monitor. Film packets are no longer an issue as PACS with it provides a filmless solution for all images. PACS can be integrated into the local area network and images from remote villages can be sent to the tertiary hospital for reporting.

PACS is an expensive investment initially but the costs can be recovered over a 5 years period. It requires a dedicated maintenance. It is important to train the doctors, technicians, nurses and other staff to use PACS effectively. Once PACS is fully operational no films are issued to patients.

PACS breaks the physical and time barriers associated with traditional film-based image retrieval, distribution and display. PACS can be linked to the internet, leading to teleradiology, the advantages of which are that images can be reviewed from home when on call, can provide linkage between two or more hospitals, outsourcing of imaging examinations in understaffed hospitals. PACS is offered by all the major medical imaging equipment manufacturers, medical IT companies and many independent software companies.